Navigating Pregnancy Challenges

Policies, Programs, and Protections

snova
New York

Obstetrics and Gynecology Advances Series

Exploring Menopause from a Multidisciplinary Perspective: Biology, Psychosocial Factors, and Clinical Insights
Nazan Yurtcu, MD, Dilay Karademir, MD and Fatih Durmuşoğlu
ISBN: 979-8-89530-001-5
eBook ISBN: 979-8-89530-108-1

Pregnancy-Associated Pelvic Girdle Pain: A Single Entity or an "Umbrella Term?"
Noa Martonovich, MD, Sharon Perlman, MD, Ophir Blickstein, MD and Ran Thein, MD
eBook ISBN: 979-8-89530-050-3

Preterm Delivery: Prevalence, Risk Factors and Related Complications
Llanos Belmonte Andujar, PhD and Ana Fuentes Rozalen, MD
ISBN: 979-8-89113-664-9
eBook ISBN: 979-8-89113-754-7

Polycystic Ovarian Syndrome (PCOS) and Our Biological Clock
Arpita Roy, PhD, Gowhar Rashid, PhD and Nihad Ashraf Khan
ISBN: 979-8-89113-100-2
eBook ISBN: 979-8-89113-212-2

Holistic Approach to Assisted Reproductive Technology
Kenan Demir and Rumeysa Göç
ISBN: 979-8-89113-017-3
eBook ISBN: 979-8-89113-064-7

More information about this series can be found at
https://novapublishers.com/product-category/series/obstetrics-and-gynecology-advances/

Javier Giles
Editor

Navigating Pregnancy Challenges

Policies, Programs, and Protections

snova
New York

Library of Congress Cataloging-in-Publication Data

ISBN: 979-8-89530-857-8 (Hardcover)
ISBN: 979-8-89530-924-7 (eBook)

Published by Nova Science Publishers, Inc. † New York

Contents

Preface

For decades, Congress has prioritized adolescent pregnancy prevention to address the public health, social, and economic challenges it poses to adolescents, their children, and society as a whole. Since the 1980s, Congress has authorized programs—administered by the U.S. Department of Health and Human Services (HHS)—designed to reduce adolescent pregnancy rates. Chapters 1 and 2 explore the evolution and status of four federally funded adolescent pregnancy prevention programs.

Adolescent childbearing carries significant social, health, and financial risks, not only for young parents but also for their families and broader communities. Despite steady declines in teen birth rates, as reported by the National Center for Health Statistics (NCHS) within the Centers for Disease Control and Prevention (CDC), the United States continues to report some of the highest rates among industrialized nations. Chapter 3 examines these teen birth trends.

Young people in the child welfare system face unique challenges, which are magnified for those who are pregnant or parenting. Chapters 4 and 5 provide strategies for caseworkers, agencies, and youth-serving professionals to better support these individuals and their families.

Federal policies also play a pivotal role in ensuring the rights and protections of pregnant individuals. Recent updates to Title IX regulations, as covered in Chapter 6, aim to eliminate discrimination against pregnant students and employees in educational institutions. Chapter 7 details the Pregnant Student Rights Act, which mandates that higher education institutions provide pregnant students with information about their rights, accommodations, and resources.

In the workplace, various federal laws safeguard employees from pregnancy-related discrimination. Chapters 8 through 11 offer an overview of key protections, such as the Pregnancy Discrimination Act (PDA), while discussing their legislative history, practical applications, and limitations. Lastly, Chapters 12 and 13 focus on resources for pregnant individuals with substance use disorders, providing valuable information for both affected individuals and the professionals who support them.

Chapter 1

Adolescent Pregnancy: Federal Prevention Programs*

Jessica Tollestrup

Summary

Congress has supported adolescent pregnancy prevention efforts for many years. These programs aim to prevent adolescent pregnancy to avert associated public health, social, and economic challenges that can affect adolescents, their children, and society. Since the 1980s, Congress has authorized—and the U.S. Department of Health and Human Services (HHS) has administered— programs with a focus on adolescent pregnancy prevention. This report assists Congress in tracking developments in four currently funded adolescent pregnancy prevention programs.

The four current programs are the *Teen Pregnancy Prevention (TPP) program*, the *Personal Responsibility Education Program (PREP)*, the *Title V Sexual Risk Avoidance Education program*, and the *General Departmental (GD) Sexual Risk Avoidance Education program*. Despite their similar names and purposes, all of these programs have different authorizing laws and funding mechanisms. Generally, the four programs serve vulnerable young people in schools, afterschool programs, community centers, and other settings. Grantees include states, nonprofits, and other entities.

The *TPP program* was initially established and funded by the FY2010 omnibus appropriations law (P.L. 111-117). Subsequent appropriations laws have also provided authority for the program and discretionary

* This is an edited, reformatted and augmented version of Congressional Research Service Publication No. R45183, dated August 22, 2024.

In: Navigating Pregnancy Challenges
Editor: Javier Giles
ISBN: 979-8-89530-857-8

funding. As required in appropriations law, the majority of TPP program grants must use evidence-based education models that have been shown to be effective in reducing adolescent pregnancy and related risk behaviors. A smaller share of funds is available for research and demonstration grants that implement innovative strategies to prevent adolescent pregnancy. The Further Continuing Appropriations Act, 2024 (P.L. 118-47), provides $101 million for the program for FY2024. Multiple HHS offices also worked together to establish the Teen Pregnancy Prevention Evidence Review process following enactment of P.L. 111-117. The review is intended to identify prevention models that have been shown to be effective based on studies since approximately the late 1990s. HHS has encouraged or required grantees for some adolescent pregnancy prevention programs to use these models. *PREP* was established under Section 513 of the Social Security Act by the Patient Protection and Affordable Care Act (ACA, P.L. 111-148) in 2010. The program receives mandatory funding and is designed to educate adolescents on both abstinence and contraception for preventing pregnancy and sexually transmitted infections, and on selected adult preparation subjects. The PREP authorizing law requires most grantees to replicate evidence-based programs that are proven to change behavior related to teen pregnancy. The Consolidated Appropriations Act, 2024 (CAA 2024, P.L. 118-42) provides $75 million for FY2024, and extends funding for the program on a prorated basis through December 31, 2024. The *Title V Sexual Risk Avoidance Education program* is authorized at Section 510 of the Social Security Act. It was formerly known as the Title V Abstinence Education Grant program, which was authorized by the 1996 welfare reform law (P.L. 104-193). The Bipartisan Budget Act of 2018 (P.L. 115-123) renamed the program and made other changes. The program focuses on implementing sexual risk avoidance, meaning voluntarily refraining from sex before marriage. Grantees may set aside some funds to conduct rigorous and evidence-based research on sexual risk avoidance. As with the PREP program, the CAA 2024 provides $75 million for FY2024, and extends funding for the program on a prorated basis through December 31, 2024.

The *GD Sexual Risk Avoidance Education program* was initially established and funded by the FY2016 omnibus appropriations law (P.L. 114-113). Subsequent appropriations laws have since provided authority for the program and discretionary funding. Grantees are to use funding for education on voluntarily refraining from nonmarital sexual activity, and they are encouraged to implement evidence-based approaches that teach the benefits associated with resisting risk behaviors. P.L. 118-47 provides FY2024 funding of $35 million for the program.

Introduction

Despite a substantial decline over the past two decades, the rate of adolescent pregnancy in the United States remains higher than that of comparable high-income countries, with persistent racial, ethnic, and geographic disparities.[1] Adolescent pregnancy has been of interest to Congress for numerous reasons, including concern about a range of associated health, social, and economic challenges that can affect adolescents, their children, and society. For instance, adolescent mothers face heightened risk of maternal complications, and their children are more likely to have poor educational, behavioral, and health outcomes.[2] In addition, adolescent pregnancy disproportionately affects certain racial and ethnic groups and selected states and insular areas.[3]

Since the 1980s, Congress and the executive branch have supported programs that focus on delaying sexual activity and preventing pregnancies among adolescents, many of which also focus on the prevention of sexually transmitted infections (STIs).[4]

Four current programs have an exclusive focus on adolescent pregnancy prevention education:[5]

---

[1] Centers for Disease Control and Prevention, *About Teen Pregnancy*, https://www.cdc.gov/reproductive-health/teen- pregnancy/index.html.

[2] Ashley M. Woodall and Anne K. Driscoll, *Racial and Ethnic Differences in Mortality Rate of Infants Born to Teen Mothers: United States, 2017–2018*, National Center for Health Statistics, Data Brief, No. 371, June 2020, https://www.cdc.gov/nchs/data/databriefs/db371-h.pdf; Emily Holcombe, Kristen Peterson, and Jennifer Manlove, *Ten Reasons to Still Keep the Focus on Teen Childbearing*, Child Trends, March 2009; Urban Institute, *Kids Having Kids: Costs and Social Consequences of Teen Pregnancy*; and Stefanie Mollborn, "Teenage Mothers Today: What we Know and How it Matters," *Child Development Perspectives*, vol. 11, no. 1 (March 2017), pp. 63-69. See also Anna Aizer, Paul Devereux, and Kjell Salvanes, "Grandparents, Moms, or Dads? Why children of teen mothers do worse in life," *Journal of Human Resources* (November 2020), pp. 1019-1052.

[3] Michelle J.K. Osterman et al., "Births: Final Data for 2022," HHS, CDC, National Center for Health Statistics (NCHS), National Vital Statistics Report, vol. 73, no. 2, April 4, 2024. See also, CRS Report R45184, *Teen Birth Trends: In Brief*.

[4] This report uses the terms *youth*, *teenagers*, *teens*, and *adolescents* interchangeably. All four programs discussed in the report generally may fund grantees that target youth aged 10 to 19, as well as older youth at-risk populations in some cases.

[5] There are several other federally funded programs that have a pregnancy prevention component and thereby may use their funds to provide pregnancy prevention information and/or contraception services to adolescents, but their focus is not exclusively on adolescents or on educational efforts. These programs include Medicaid Family Planning (Title XIX of the Social Security Act), Title X Family Planning, the Maternal and Child Health block grant (Title V of the Social Security Act), the Temporary Assistance for Needy Families (TANF) block grant (Title IV-A of the Social Security Act), and selected other programs administered by the U.S. Department of Health and Human Services (HHS).

- the Teen Pregnancy Prevention (TPP) program, which is authorized on an annual basis under the Departments of Labor, Health and Human Services, Education, and related agencies (LHHS) appropriations;
- the Personal Responsibility Education Program (PREP), which is authorized under Title V of the Social Security Act, and was most recently reauthorized through FY2023, under Title III, Division CC of the Consolidated Appropriations Act, 2021 (CAA 2021, P.L. 116-260);
- the Title V Sexual Risk Avoidance Education program, which is authorized under Title V of the Social Security Act, and was most recently reauthorized through FY2023, under Title III, Division CC of the CAA 2021; and
- the Sexual Risk Avoidance Education program, which is authorized on an annual basis under the LHHS appropriations, and is sometimes referred to as the General Departmental (GD) Sexual Risk Avoidance Education program.

This report refers to the latter two programs as the Title V Sexual Risk Avoidance Education program and the GD Sexual Risk Avoidance Education program, respectively, to avoid confusion.[6] The four programs are administered in the U.S. Department of Health and Human Services (HHS). The TPP program was administered by the Office of Adolescent Health (OAH) until it was subsumed under the Office of Population Affairs (OPA) in the Office of the Assistant Secretary for Health (OASH) in June 2019.[7] (The

[6] Both of these programs generally require that grantees focus on teaching abstinence before marriage. The programs can be distinguished in a few ways. The Title V Sexual Risk Avoidance Education program is authorized at Section 510 (Title V) of the Social Security Act. It was formerly known as the Title V Abstinence Education Grant program, which was authorized by the 1996 welfare reform law (P.L. 104-193). The Bipartisan Budget Act of 2018 (BBA 2018, P.L. 115-123) renamed the program and specified new program requirements on financial allotments, educational elements, research and data, and evaluations. The General Departmental (GD) Sexual Risk Avoidance Education program was established and first funded by the FY2016 omnibus appropriations laws and has since been funded by subsequent appropriations laws. The appropriations laws have provided some detail about how the Sexual Risk Avoidance Education program is to be carried out. Because it is funded under the General Departmental Management account in appropriations law, HHS often refers to the program as the "General Departmental" Sexual Risk Avoidance Education program.

[7] The conference report (H.Rept. 111-366) accompanying the FY2010 appropriations law (P.L. 111-117) directed the HHS Secretary to establish an Office of Adolescent Health (OAH) responsible for implementing and administering the Teen Pregnancy Prevention (TPP)

footnotes of the report continue to reference publications that were authored by OAH.) The three other programs are administered by the Family and Youth Services Bureau (FYSB) in HHS's Administration for Children and Families (ACF).

This report provides background on the role of Congress and the executive branch in preventing adolescent pregnancy. It then focuses on the four adolescent pregnancy prevention programs, examining the types of grants they provide as well as related funding, requirements, and research and evaluation activities. *Table A-1* summarizes key programmatic information and allows for comparisons across the programs. *Table B-1* indicates whether the states and insular areas, or entities within those jurisdictions, receive funding under each of the four programs. The report accompanies CRS Report R45184, *Teen Birth Trends: In Brief*; and CRS In Focus IF10877, *Federal Teen Pregnancy Prevention Programs*.

Federal Approaches to Adolescent Pregnancy Prevention

The federal government has long played a role in educating adolescents and the general public about preventing pregnancy and STIs. This has involved public awareness campaigns; providing public health services, including information and access to contraceptives; publishing materials about STIs; and funding organizations to provide sexual education. The federal approach to adolescent pregnancy prevention has often reflected prevailing public views about sexuality and the role that the federal government should play in the private lives of its citizens.[8]

Since the early 1980s, the federal government has supported programs that have an exclusive focus on preventing adolescent pregnancy.[9] Discussion

program. The report also directed OAH to coordinate its efforts with ACF, CDC, and other appropriate offices and operating divisions in HHS. See also the Statement of Organization, Functions, and Delegations of Authority filed in the *Federal Register* on April 12, 2019, explaining the new organizational structure for the OPA that would include the TPP program (84 *Federal Register* 14951).

[8] Alexandra M. Lord, *Condom Nation: the U.S. Government's Sex Education Campaign from World War I to the Internet* (Baltimore: Johns Hopkins University Press, 2010), pp. 1-24, 115-137, 162-186.

[9] Three programs are no longer funded: the Adolescent Family Life (AFL) program, the Community-Based Abstinence Education (CBAE) program, and the Competitive Abstinence-Only program. The AFL program was established in 1981 and funded through FY2001, with appropriations ranging from \$1.4 million to \$30.4 million annually. The program focused on issues of adolescent sexuality, pregnancy, and parenting, and in 1998

about these programs has often focused on the type of approaches to pregnancy prevention they should take. Some policymakers and other stakeholders in the adolescent pregnancy prevention field have contended that adolescents should not engage in sex before marriage to avoid unplanned pregnancies and protect against STIs.

Further, they support the idea that adolescents need to hear a single, unambiguous message that sex outside of marriage is harmful to their physical and emotional health.[10] This approach is sometimes referred to as abstinence-only, and more recently as sexual risk avoidance.

Other stakeholders have prioritized an approach that provides broad information to adolescents to help them make informed decisions about whether to engage in sex, and about using contraceptives if they do.[11] They contend that such an approach allows young people to make choices regarding abstinence, gives them the information they need to set relationship limits and resist peer pressure, and provides them with information on the use of contraceptives and the prevention of STIs.

Congress has authorized and provided funding for programs that take one or both of these approaches to preventing adolescent pregnancy. Of the current programs, the Title V Sexual Risk Avoidance Education and the GD Sexual Risk Avoidance Education programs predominantly focus on abstaining from premarital sex. The PREP program requires most grantees to place "substantial emphasis on both abstinence and contraception for the prevention of pregnancy among youth and STIs."[12] TPP grantees may use either or both approaches.[13]

---

it began incorporating abstinence-only education. The CBAE program was supported from FY2001 through FY2009, with funding ranging from $20 million to $108.9 million annually. The program provided competitive grants to public and private entities to develop and implement abstinence-only education programs for adolescents aged 12 through 18 in communities nationwide. Following CBAE, the Competitive Abstinence-Only program supported similar types of grants with an exclusive focus on abstinence education. It was funded from FY2012 through FY2015, with appropriations of $4.7 million to $10 million annually.

[10] See, for example, U.S. House of Representatives, Committee on Energy and Commerce, *The Policy Paper Series: Transforming Ideas Into Solutions, vol. 1, issue 2*, "A Better Approach to Teenage Pregnancy Prevention-Sexual Risk Avoidance," July 2012.

[11] HHS, CDC, Dear Colleague Letter by Thomas R. Frieden, Director, January 14, 2011. Dr. Frieden served under the Obama Administration from May 2009 to January 2017.

[12] Section 513(b)(2)(4) of the Social Security Act.

[13] Amy Feldman Farb and Amy L. Margolis, "The Teen Pregnancy Prevention Program (2010-2015): Synthesis of Impact Findings," *American Journal of Public Health*, vol. 106, no. 51 (September 2016) (hereinafter, Amy Feldman Farb and Amy L. Margolis, "The Teen Pregnancy Prevention Program (2010-2015): Synthesis of Impact Findings").

Surveys measuring public opinion about adolescent sexual activity and contraceptive use show a range of perspectives, possibly due to differences in the design of the survey questions and the population surveyed. Based on one nationally representative survey in 2017 by Power to Decide, an organization focused on preventing unplanned pregnancy, most adults believe that teens should receive more information about abstinence and contraception, as well as protection from STIs.[14] However, in 2022 Pew Research in its American Trends Panel found that most parents of K-12 students (59%) reported "they would prefer that their children learn [in school] that there are methods of contraception that are safe and effective ways to prevent unintended pregnancy and STIs; 22% would rather their children learn that abstaining from sex is the only safe and effective method to prevent unintended pregnancy and STIs, and 18% say their children shouldn't learn about this in school." The views of respondents differed somewhat based on their political affiliation and the age of their children.[15]

The Use of Evidence-Based Models

Two of the current adolescent pregnancy programs, TPP and PREP, reflect government-wide efforts beginning in the George W. Bush Administration and extending into the Obama Administration, to expand effective social

---

[14] SSRS, an independent research organization, conducted the poll for Power to Decide, which generally supports providing youth with information so they can make informed decisions about whether, when, and under what circumstances to get pregnant and have a child (Power to Decide was formerly known as the National Campaign to Prevent Teen and Unplanned Pregnancy). The poll involved a nationally representative telephone survey of approximately 1,000 adults in the United States that asked, "Do you believe that teens should receive more information about abstinence or postponing sex [8% supported this view], birth control and STI protection [10% supported this view], or both [79% supported this view]?" See Power to Decide, "Survey Says: Support for Birth Control," January 2017.

[15] The Pew American Trends Panel is a nationally representative panel of randomly selected U.S. adults who serve as a survey panel and agree to take multiple surveys. In this survey, panel members who are parents of K-12 students were asked whether they would prefer their children learn in school that "there are methods of contraception that are safe and effective ways to prevent unintended pregnancy and STIs" [59% supported this view], "abstinence is the only safe and effective way to prevent unintended pregnancy and sexually transmitted infections" [22%], and "children should not learn about this in school" [18%]. See Pew Research Center, "Parents Differ Sharply by Part Over What Their K-12 Children Should Learn in School," October 26, 2022, https://www.pewresearch.org/social-trends/2022/10/26/parents-differ-sharply-by-party-over-what-their-k-12-children-should-learn-in-school/.

interventions and eliminate those that are ineffective.[16] The two programs use a "tiered evidence" approach, wherein some current grantees employ adolescent pregnancy prevention models that are effective based on rigorous evaluation while other grantees develop and rigorously evaluate new or innovative approaches aimed at reducing teen pregnancy. In addition, although the Title V SRAE and GD SRAE programs do not use this same framework, recent grant announcements have required that grantees use "evidence-based" interventions.[17]

Evaluation requirements and projects specific to each of the adolescent pregnancy prevention programs in this report are discussed in their respective report sections. Two broad-based efforts associated with these programs that are intended to inform the field as a whole are summarized below.[18]

Teen Pregnancy Prevention Evidence Review

Following enactment of the FY2010 omnibus appropriations law (P.L. 111-117), which authorized the TPP program and required it to use models that are proven effective through rigorous evaluation in reducing teen pregnancy and related outcomes, multiple HHS offices worked together to establish the Teen Pregnancy Prevention Evidence Review (TPPER) process.

Broadly, the TPPER systematically reviews research on teen pregnancy prevention to identify programs that have an impact on reducing (1) teen

---

[16] Evelyn M. Kappeler and Amy Feldman Farb, "Historical Context for the Creation of the Office of Adolescent Health and the Teen Pregnancy Prevention Program," *Journal of Adolescent Health*, vol. 54, no. 3 (March 2014) (hereinafter, Evelyn M. Kappeler and Amy Feldman Farb, "Historical Context for the Creation of the Office of Adolescent Health and the Teen Pregnancy Prevention Program"). In June 2019, the Office of Adolescent Health was subsumed under the Office of Population Affairs (OPA). See also, Ron Haskins and Greg Margolis, *Show Me the Evidence: Obama's Fight for Rigor and Results in Social Policy*, Brookings Institution Press, Washington, DC, 2014; and Heather Fish et al., *What Works for Adolescent Sexual and Reproductive Health: Lessons from Experimental Evaluations of Programs and Interventions*, Child Trends, publication no. 2014-64, December 2014.

[17] "Evidence-based" is defined as "interventions, strategies, approaches, and/or program models that have been evaluated using rigorous evaluation design such as randomized controlled or high-quality, quasi-experimental trials, and that have demonstrated positive impacts for youth, families, and communities." See HHS, ACF, FYSB, *Title V Competitive Sexual Risk Avoidance Education (SRAE)*, Funding Opportunity Announcement and Instruction, HHS-2024-ACF-ACYF-TS-0040, 2024; and HHS, ACF, FYSB, *General Departmental Sexual Risk Avoidance Education (GD-SRAE)*, Funding Opportunity Announcement and Instructions. HHS-2024-ACF-ACYF-SR-0041, 2024.

[18] This section does not address other surveillance or research activities, such as the CDC Youth Risk Behavior Surveillance System or the National Vital Statistics System.

pregnancy and STIs and (2) sexual risk behaviors.[19] The TPPER is managed by the Assistant Secretary for Planning and Evaluation (ASPE) in collaboration with FYSB within the Administration for Children and Families (ACF), and the former Office of Adolescent Health (OAH) within the Office of the Assistant Secretary for Health (OASH). Despite the connection to the TPP program, the review is intended to more broadly inform the adolescent pregnancy prevention field.

The TPPER was initially active from 2010 to 2019, and identified teen pregnancy prevention models that were shown to be effective based on studies from the prior 30 years.[20] After a pause in activity during the Trump Administration, funding to restart the review was set aside as part of FY2022 appropriations, and HHS issued a call for new studies to be submitted for review.[21] The latest findings were released in 2023.[22]

The TPPER uses a systematic process to identify studies with statistically significant impacts on at least one of five outcomes: (1) sexual activity, (2) number of sexual partners, (3) contraceptive use, (4) STIs or HIV, and (5) pregnancies. The review specifically examines studies on U.S. youth who are ages 19 and younger; however, the review examines studies from programs that are delivered in various settings (e.g., one-on-one educational sessions, or classroom-based curricula) and from programs that may use a range of methods or approaches (e.g., skill-building sessions, psycho-social interventions).

---

[19] Office of the Assistant Secretary for Health: Office of Population Affairs, *Updated Findings from the HHS Teen Pregnancy Prevention Evidence Review (TPPER): What is the TPPER?*, https://opa.hhs.gov/research-evaluation/teen-pregnancy-prevention-program-evaluations/tpp-evidence-review.

[20] When it was initially established, HHS contracted with Mathematica Policy Research, Inc., a social policy research organization, to review studies of teen pregnancy prevention programs. Such research was identified through a call for studies and review of journals, conference proceedings, and websites for research and policy organizations. See Juliet Lugo-Gil et al., *Updated Findings from the HHS Teen Pregnancy Prevention Evidence Review: August 2015 through October 2016*, Mathematica Policy Research, for HHS, ASPE, April 2018.

[21] See page H2684 of the joint explanatory statement accompanying FY2022 LHHS appropriations (*Congressional Record,* vol. 168, no. 42, book IV [March 9, 2022]); in reestablishing the TPPER, HHS contracted with Mathematica Policy Research to lead the review of the submitted studies (HHS, *HHS Teen Pregnancy Prevention (TPP) Evidence Review Call for Studies*, https://youth.gov/sites/default/files/2022-03/2022_TPPER_Call_for_Papers.pdf).

[22] HHS, OPA, OASH, "Updated Findings from the HHS Teen Pregnancy Prevention Evidence Review (TPPER)," July 5, 2023, https://opa.hhs.gov/research-evaluation/teen-pregnancy-prevention-program-evaluations/tpp-evidence-review.

Additionally, the studies must evaluate impacts of programs or program components using randomized controlled trials (RCTs) or quasi-experimental impact study designs.[23] For the studies that meet these initial criteria, reviewers assign each one a rating of high, moderate, or low quality based on the study design, the degree of attrition, whether the study controls for differences between the treatment and comparison groups, and whether it meets certain other criteria that minimize the risk of study bias.[24]

The TPPER has been updated multiple times since its initial establishment in 2010. The first review covered research released from 1989 through January 2010 and identified 28 effective program models. Subsequent reviews were conducted on an annual or biannual basis through 2018, and again through May 2023, to incorporate recent research, including newly available evidence for programs that were previously reviewed. Cumulatively through 2023, TPPER reviews have identified 52 evidence-based program models.[25]

The most recent TPPER includes program models that approach adolescent pregnancy from different frameworks. HHS categorizes the evidence-based models based on certain key features. For example, three of the identified models use a sexual risk avoidance approach; other models focus, for example, on health relationships, positive youth development, or sexual health education. The models also differ based on their outcomes, settings (e.g., schools, clinics, homes, communities), session length and duration over time, and target population (e.g., intended race/ethnicity, age or grade level, gender, sexually active youth).[26]

---

[23] RCTs involve assigning individuals to two groups—an intervention group and a control group—using a random process (e.g., a lottery) to compare outcomes across these groups. Under ideal conditions, this can help to explain whether an intervention, like abstinence education, is effective because youth in both the program and control groups were similar in all respects except for their access to the program. Quasi-experimental designs refer to studies that attempt to estimate a treatment's impact on a group of subjects but, in contrast to RCTs, do not have random assignment to treatment and control groups. Some quasi-experiments are controlled studies (i.e., with a control group), but others lack a control group.

[24] See Mathematica Policy Research, *Identifying Programs That Impact Teen Pregnancy, Sexually Transmitted Infections, and Associated Sexual Risk Behaviors*, Review Protocol, version 7.0, for HHS, ASPE, October 2023.

[25] HHS, OPA, OASH, "Updated Findings from the HHS Teen Pregnancy Prevention Evidence Review (TPPER," July 5, 2023, https://opa.hhs.gov/research-evaluation/teen-pregnancy-prevention-program-evaluations/tpp-evidence-review.

[26] HHS, OASH, OPA, "Find and Compare Programs," https://youth.gov/evidence-innovation/tpper/compare-programs.

Additional Evaluations of Teenage Pregnancy Prevention Approaches

HHS has developed additional research on adolescent pregnancy prevention interventions through annual transfers under Section 241 of the Public Health Service Act (PHSA) of approximately $4.5 million to $6.8 million from FY2011-FY2024.[27] These Section 241 transfers are directed in annual LHHS appropriations acts under a provision in the General Departmental Management account, the same account that funds the TPP program. The purpose of these funds is "to carry out evaluations (including longitudinal evaluations) of teenage pregnancy prevention approaches." For FY2025, these evaluation supports include

- two research-to-practice centers to develop and disseminate research-informed practice resources for professionals who work with youth involved in the child welfare and/or justice systems, youth experiencing homelessness, and disconnected youth (also referred to as opportunity youth), and to develop resources for providing trauma-informed and inclusive care;
- research grants that examine the settings and youth characteristics to determine under what conditions TPP programs are most and least effective, and the determining factors that prevent and reduce disparities in sexual health outcomes;
- rigorous evaluation training and technical assistance to TPP program grantees conducting research and evaluation;
- collection and analysis of program performance measures for monitoring, program improvement, and reporting;
- multiple research projects with the goals of identifying, measuring, and evaluating the effectiveness of core components of TPP programs; and
- in partnership with the Office of the Assistant Secretary for Planning and Evaluation and the Administration for Children and Families, the HHS TPP Evidence Review to build a collective understanding of the program models that have been rigorously evaluated and shown to

[27] Section 241 of the PHSA provides authority for HHS to transfer funds between PHSA accounts to conduct evaluations of the implementation and effectiveness of public health programs. LHHS appropriations acts commonly establish requirements in addition to those in statute. These include directing specific amounts of funding transferred pursuant to Section 241 to selected HHS programs.

reduce teen pregnancy, sexually transmitted infections, or associated sexual risk behaviors.[28]

Teen Pregnancy Prevention (TPP) Program

The Consolidated Appropriations Act, FY2010 (P.L. 111-117) established and provided annual discretionary funding for the Teen Pregnancy Prevention program (TPP).[29] The OAH administered the program until it was subsumed under the OPA in June 2019.[30]

The TPP program has been funded via the appropriations process through FY2024. Funding has ranged from approximately $98 million to $110 million annually. As discussed above, the TPP program primarily provides funds for evidence-based programs and/or programs that show promise toward reducing adolescent and young adult pregnancy, including those that focus on sexual risk avoidance and/or use of contraceptives (see the "The Use of Evidence-Based Models" section).

Generally, the appropriations laws have stated that funding should be competitively awarded. They have further specified that no more than 10% of TPP funding may be used for training and technical assistance, outreach, and other program support. Of the remaining amount, the appropriations laws have stated the following:

- 75% is for grants to replicate programs that have been proven through rigorous evaluation to be effective in reducing teenage pregnancy,

---

[28] HHS, *Fiscal Year 2025 Justification of Estimates for Appropriations Committees for General Departmental Management,* pp. 132-133, https://www.hhs.gov/sites/default/files/fy-2025-gdm-cj.pdf. See also Evelyn M. Kappeler and Amy Feldman Farb, "Historical Context for the Creation of the Office of Adolescent Health and the Teen Pregnancy Prevention Program."

[29] The program had been proposed as part of President Obama's FY2010 budget to replace the abstinence education program known as the Community-Based Abstinence Education (CBAE) program. See HHS, *Fiscal Year 2010 Justification of Estimates for Appropriations Committees for Administration for Children and Families*, pp. 55-56 and 74. The CBAE program was funded from FY2001 through FY2009.

[30] The conference report (H.Rept. 111-366) accompanying the FY2010 appropriations law (P.L. 111-117) directed the HHS Secretary to establish an Office of Adolescent Health responsible for implementing and administering the TPP program. The report also directed OAH to coordinate its efforts with ACF, CDC, and other appropriate offices and operating divisions in HHS.

behavioral factors underlying teen pregnancy, or other related risk factors. HHS has referred to these as "Tier 1" grants.

- 25% is for research and demonstration grants to develop, replicate, and refine additional models and innovative strategies for reducing teenage pregnancy. HHS refers to these as "Tier 2" grants.

Appropriation laws also have specified that funds must be used for "age appropriate" and "medically accurate" programs that reduce teen pregnancy. HHS has expanded on these terms and has established eligibility and other requirements via funding announcements and other publications. In 2023, "age appropriateness" was defined by HHS in the funding announcement for the most recent Tier 1 cohort as, "Ensures that topics, messages, and teaching methods are suitable to particular ages or age groups of children and adolescents, based on developing cognitive, emotional, and behavioral capacity typical for the age or age group." "Medical accuracy" was defined as "verified or supported by the weight of research conducted in compliance with accepted scientific methods; and published in peer-reviewed journals, where applicable or comprising information that leading professional organizations and agencies with relevant expertise in the field recognize as accurate, objective, and complete."[31]

A range of public and private entities have been eligible to apply for TPP funding. Such entities include nonprofit and for-profit organizations, universities and colleges, faith- and community- based organizations, hospitals, and research institutions, among other entities.

---

[31] HHS, OASH, OPA, *Advancing Equity in Adolescent Health through Evidence-Based Teen Pregnancy Prevention Programs and Services*, AH-TP1-23-001, 2023. Other definitions have been used by HHS over the years. For example, in the funding opportunity announcement for 2020, "age appropriate" was defined as content "appropriate for the general developmental and social maturity of the targeted age group. The ability to cognitively understand a concept is not evidence that the concept is age appropriate." For content to be "medically accurate," that "information [would] be referenced to peer reviewed publications by educational, scientific, governmental, or health organizations." HHS, OASH, OPA, *Optimally Changing the Map for Teen Pregnancy Prevention (Tier 1), Funding Opportunity Announcement and Application Instructions*, AH-TP1-20-001, 2020.

Tier 1 Grants

The TPP grants have supported multiple cohorts of Tier 1 grantees since FY2010. The first cohort was funded for FY2010-FY2014.[32] The second cohort had multiple rounds of funding due to the early termination of the first round of funding in 2017 (initially awarded for FY2015-FY2020);[33] an additional round of funding was later awarded for FY2019-FY2021.[34] A third cohort of Tier 1 funding was funded for FY2020-FY2023[35] and FY2021-FY2023.[36] The fourth (and most recent) cohort of Tier 1 awards covers the period of FY2023-FY2028, contingent on the future availability of funds.[37]

This fourth cohort of Tier 1 grantees—Advancing Equity in Adolescent Health through Evidence- Based Teen Pregnancy Prevention Program and Services—supports 53 grantees in 25 states and Puerto Rico.[38] These grants

---

[32] HHS, OASH, OAH, *The Teen Pregnancy Prevention (TPP) Program: Performance in the First Five Years,* April 2016.

[33] In spring 2017, HHS sent notices to all 84 TPP grantees funded in the second round informing them that their expected five-year projects would end in June or September 2018 instead of June or September 2020. In addition, five organizations that provided technical assistance to the grantees were informed that their expected five-year grant period ended in June 2017 instead of June 2022. This included all of the TPP grant types. In response, eight lawsuits were filed in February and March 2018 on behalf of all the grantees except for the Tier 2C grantees (discussed later in this report). From April to June 2018, five of the lawsuits were decided in favor of the grantees, including a class action lawsuit that applied to the three remaining lawsuits. In September 2018, HHS discontinued funding for two of the three Tier 2C grantees, which were not included in the original litigation. That same month, one of the Tier 2C grantees, Promundo, filed a separate lawsuit. The court dismissed this grantee's claim for FY2018 funding because the funding was no longer available for obligation.

[34] HHS, OASH, Office of Population Affairs (OPA), "OPA Awards $13.5 Million in Grants to Replicate Teenage Pregnancy Programs," July 11, 2019, https://www.hhs.gov/ash/oah/news/news-releases/2019-tpp-tier1-award-grantees/ index.html.

[35] HHS, OASH, OPA, "OPA Awards $56.3 Million in Grants to Replicate Effective Teenage Pregnancy Prevention Programs," June 30, 2020, https://opa.hhs.gov/about/news/grant-award-announcements/opa-awards-563-million- grants-replicate-effective-teenage.

[36] HHS, OASH, OPA, "OPA Awards $12.6 Million in Grants to Replicate Effective Teenage Pregnancy Prevention Programs," June 28, 2021, https://opa.hhs.gov/about/news/grant-award-announcements/opa-awards-12-million-grants- replicate-effective-teenage#:~:text=The%20Office%20of%20Population%20Affairs,a%20two%2Dyear%20project%20period.

[37] HHS, OASH, OPA, "HHS Announces $68 Million for Teen Pregnancy Prevention Opportunities," June 23, 2023, https://www.hhs.gov/about/news/2023/06/23/hhs-announces-69-million-for-teen-pregnancy-prevention- opportunities.html.

[38] HHS, OASH, OPA, *About the Teen Pregnancy Prevention Program,* https://opa.hhs.gov/grant-programs/teen-pregnancy-prevention-program/about-tpp-program; and HHS, OASH, OPA, Current Teen Pregnancy Prevention Grant Recipients, https://opa.hhs.gov/grant-programs/teen-pregnancy-prevention-program/tpp-grant-recipients/current-tpp-grant-recipients.

seek to scale up effective programs that have been proven through rigorous evaluation to reduce teenage pregnancy, behavioral risk factors underlying teenage pregnancy, or other associated risk factors. *Rigorous evaluation* refers to results that come from robust evaluation designs, particularly experiments or quasi-experiments.[39]

In general, Tier 1 grantees must implement their models consistent with the original evidence- based model listed in the TPP Evidence Review and have minimal adaptations (e.g., changing names). In the application materials for the most recent Tier 1 grantee cohort, HHS defined "evidence-based approaches" as those "that have been proven effective through rigorous evaluation to reduce teenage pregnancy, behavioral risk factors underlying teenage pregnancy, or other associated risk factors."[40] HHS further emphasized the importance of grantees using materials accompanying the evidence-based programs that are "age appropriate, medically accurate, culturally and linguistically appropriate, trauma-informed, and inclusive of all youth."[41]

Grantee Profile: Partners in Social Research, LLC (PSR)

PSR aims to reduce teen pregnancy by partnering with schools, community stakeholders, afterschool programs, a teen clinic in the city of New Britain, CT, and statewide programs for youth with child welfare involvement to select and implement evidence-based teen pregnancy prevention programs. This project will establish a Teen Pregnancy Prevention Advisory, which will work in coordination with the New Britain Prevention Council to create and sustain a robust network of partners: community stakeholders, educators, health providers, families and caregivers, LGBTQ+ advocates, and youth leaders as equal decisionmakers in this effort. The programs will be implemented in middle schools (grades 6-8), high schools, alternative schools, community and afterschool programs, clinics, and in child welfare settings. All materials disseminated to youth will be reviewed at least annually to ensure that they are medically accurate, age-appropriate,

[39] HHS, OAH, *Teenage Pregnancy Prevention: Replication of Evidence-based Programs Funding Opportunity Announcement and Application Instructions*, 2010.

[40] HHS, OASH, OPA, *Advancing Equity in Adolescent Health through Evidence-Based Teen Pregnancy Prevention Programs and Services*, *Funding Opportunity Announcement and Application Instructions,* AH-TP1-23-001, 2023.

[41] Ibid.

culturally and linguistically appropriate, trauma-informed, and inclusive of all youth. The project will not only give young people the tools to prevent teen pregnancy and sexually transmitted infections (STIs), but it will also mobilize the community to build a network of youth-friendly services to meet young people's social, physical, psychological, and financial needs.

Source: HHS, OASH, OPA, Current Teen Pregnancy Prevention Grant Recipients: Advancing Equity in Adolescent Health through Evidence-Based Teen Pregnancy Prevention Program and Services (TPP23 Tier 1) – 2023-2028.

Note: This report includes examples of grantees recently funded under the four teen pregnancy prevention programs. The grantees were selected by CRS based on information available on the HHS website or provided via correspondence with HHS. Collectively, the grantees described in the report are intended to represent all regions of the country and are included for illustrative purposes only.

Tier 2 Grants

As with Tier 1 grantees, HHS has funded multiple cohorts of Tier 2 grants over the years, with the different announcements within a cohort sometimes referred to as "phases." The first cohort of grantees was funded for FY2010-2014. The second cohort of grantees was funded for FY2015-FY2020[42] with some additional grants later awarded and funded for FY2018-FY2020.[43] The third cohort of Tier 2 grants was funded for FY2020-FY2023 and separated into two phases: TPP Innovation and Impact Networks (Tier 2; TPP20 Innovation Networks),[44] and Phase 2 Rigorous Evaluation of Promising TPP

[42] HHS, OASH, OAH, Supporting and Enabling Early Innovation to Advance Adolescent Health and Prevent Teen Pregnancy (Tier 2A), Funding Opportunity Announcement and Application Instructions, AH-TP2-15-001, 2015; HHS, OASH, OAH, Rigorous Evaluation of New or Innovative Approaches to Prevent Teen Pregnancy Tier 2B), Funding Opportunity Announcement and Application Instructions, AH-TP2-15-002, 2015; and HHS, CDC, Effectiveness of Teen Pregnancy Prevention Programs Designed Specifically for Young Males [Tier 2C], Funding Opportunity Announcement, RFA-DP-15-007, 2015.

[43] HHS, OASH, OPA, Phase I New and Innovative Strategies (Tier 2) to Prevent Teenage Pregnancy and Promote Health Adolescence, Funding Opportunity Announcement, AH-TP2-18-001, 2018. According to the funding announcement, the objective for Phase II was to build on the results achieved in Phase I and is limited to successful Phase I grantees.

[44] HHS, OASH, OPA, "OPA Awards $19.2 Million in Grants to Develop Innovation and Impact Networks to Prevent Teen Pregnancy and Achieve Optimal Health," July 14, 2020,

Interventions (Tier 2 Phase 2; TPP Rigorous Evaluation).[45] The fourth (and most recent) cohort of Tier 2 grants was awarded for FY2023-FY2028, contingent on the future availability of funds; as with the third cohort, these grants are distinguished by the phase of evidence-building that they are intended to support. The Adolescent Sexual Health Innovation Hubs and Rigorous Evaluation Cooperative Agreements support six grantees in four states as they carry out programs that will "develop, refine, and test additional models and innovative strategies."[46] In addition, TPP Rigorous Evaluation Cooperative Agreements were awarded to 12 grantees across nine states and the District of Columbia to continue the work of previous Phase 2 grants.[47]

TPP Evaluation Activities

Since the early years of the TPP program, HHS has supported numerous program evaluations to determine which models and approaches are effective. These evaluations have shown a range of results, with many identifying programs with positive impacts on teen pregnancy-related outcomes. For example, for the first cohort of grantees HHS supported a federal effort to conduct 41 evaluations.[48] Of these, 12 showed a positive impact in at least one teen pregnancy-related outcome. Another 16 had no impacts (one of these also had a negative impact), and 13 had inconclusive results. Some of the evaluations were inconclusive because of high attrition, weak contrasts between the treatment and control groups, a failure to meet HHS's research standards, or other reasons.[49] In the intervening years since the inception of

---

https://opa.hhs.gov/about/news/grant-award-announcements/opa-awards-192-million-grants-develop-innovation-and-impact.

[45] HHS, OASH, OPA, "OPA Awards $3.7 Million in Grants to Conduct Evaluation of Promising Interventions to Prevent Teen Pregnancy and Achieve Optimal Health," July 14, 2020, https://opa.hhs.gov/about/news/grant-award-announcements/opa-awards-37-million-grants-conduct-evaluation-promising.

[46] HHS, OASH, "HHS Awards $23 Million to Support Evidence-Based Teen Pregnancy Prevention Programs," August 25, 2023, https://www.hhs.gov/about/news/2023/08/25/hhs-awards-23-million-support-evidence-based-teen- pregnancy-prevention.html.

[47] Ibid.

[48] This included 19 Tier 1 evaluations of 10 evidence-based models identified as part of the Teen Pregnancy Prevention Evidence Review. The evaluations also included 22 studies of Tier 2 grantees, which were expected to implement new or innovative models to improve teen pregnancy-related outcomes.

[49] Amy Feldman Farb and Amy L. Margolis, "The Teen Pregnancy Prevention Program (2010-2015): Synthesis of Impact Findings."

the program, HHS has continued to fund evaluations of TPP program effectiveness; some of these are summarized below.

In general, the Tier 1 TPP grants across all cohorts have required some type of evaluation for at least some grantees, although these requirements have varied. For the first cohort (FY2010- FY2014), all Tier 1 grantees that received a specified level of funding were required to be evaluated, and all grantees regardless of funding level were required to monitor and report on program implementation and outcomes according to performance measures.[50] The second (FY2015-FY2021) and third (FY2020-FY2023) cohorts did not distinguish between grantees by level of funding, and instead expected that all grantees evaluate the implementation of their programs.[51] The fourth cohort (FY2023-FY2028) grantees are to monitor and report on their program impacts, but were directed not to use funds for a rigorous impact evaluation.[52]

With regard to the Tier 2 TPP grantees, as the general purpose of these grants is to establish an evidence base for new approaches, they have all generally required some type of evaluation. However, most cohorts have split these grantees into phases, with the first phase supporting interventions that are in the early stage of development, and the second phase supporting interventions that are ready for rigorous evaluation.[53] In such cases, the type of evaluation expected in each phase has differed. For example, Phase 1 of the third cohort (FY2020-FY2023) required that the grantee test and evaluate interventions at different stages of development. In the funding opportunity announcement, HHS stated, "It is expected that some interventions will move between testing and development, evolving throughout the course of the project, and it is expected that interventions will be refined based on learnings. Grantees should use testing and evaluation methods appropriate for the stage of intervention development, collecting and analyzing data to make changes

---

[50] HHS, OAH, "Teenage Pregnancy Prevention: Replication of Evidence-based Programs (Tier 1)," Funding Opportunity Announcement, OPHS/OAHTPP Tier1-2010, 2010.

[51] HHS, OAH, "Capacity Building to Support Replication of Evidence-Based TPP Programs (Tier 1B), AH-TP1-15- 001, 2015; HHS, OAH, "Phase I Replicating Programs (Tier 1) Effective in the Promotion of Healthy Adolescence and the Reduction of Teenage Pregnancy and Associated Risk Behaviors," AH-TP1-18-001, 2018; and HHS, OAH, OPA, "Optimally Change the Map of Teen Pregnancy through Replication of Programs Proven Effective (Optimally Changing the Map for Teen Pregnancy Prevention – Tier 1)," AH-TP1-20-001, 2020.

[52] HHS, OAH, OPA, "Advancing Equity in Adolescent Health through Evidence-Based Teen Pregnancy Prevention Programs and Services" AH-TP1-23-001, 2023.

[53] See, for example, HHS, OAH, "Supporting and Enabling Early Innovation to Advance Adolescent Health and Prevent Teen Pregnancy (Tier 2A), AH-TP2-15-001, 2015; HHS, OAH, "Rigorous Evaluation of New or Innovative Approaches to Prevent Teen Pregnancy (Tier 2B)," AH-TP2-15-002, 2015.

and assess impacts."[54] In contrast, Phase 2 funding was provided specifically to support more developed programs where rigorous evaluation was appropriate.[55] Similarly, the fourth cohort (FY2023-FY2028) of Tier 2 grants were awarded in two separate funding streams: grants for "innovation hubs" to support early evaluation efforts for developing programs, and grants for interventions that are ready to be rigorously evaluated.[56]

The MITRE Corporation, which currently operates the Health Federally Funded Research and Development Center (FFRDC) under contract with the Centers for Medicare and Medicaid Services (CMS), was awarded funding for FY2017 and FY2018 to test and replicate meaningful ways to improve programs related to teen pregnancy prevention under the Teen Pregnancy Prevention Study.[57] MITRE subcontracted with multiple entities to carry out activities under the contract. The project included several activities, including revising SMARTool,[58] evaluating organizations that implement sexual risk avoidance education curricula that align with SMARTool, and developing and testing surveys of youth with key topics from SMARTool.[59]

For the third cohort of TPP grantees, in addition to the required individual grantee evaluations, OPA contracted with Abt Associates and its partners, Decision Information Resources and Data Soapbox, to evaluate how the Tier 1 (Optimally Changing the Map for Teen Pregnancy Prevention) and Tier 2

[54] HHS, OAH, OPA, "Tier 2 Innovation and Impact Network Grants: Achieving Optimal Health and Preventing Teen Pregnancy in Key Priority Areas" AH-TP2-20-002, 2020.

[55] HHS, OAH, OPA, "Teen Pregnancy Prevention (TPP) Tier 2, Phase II Rigorous Evaluation of Promising Interventions" AH-TP2-20-001, 2020.

[56] HHS, OAH, OPA, "Teen Pregnancy Prevention Tier 2 Adolescent Sexual Health Innovation Hubs" AH-TP2-23-002, 2023; and HHS, OAH, OPA, "Teen Pregnancy Prevention Tier 2 Rigorous Evaluation Cooperative Agreements" AH- TP2-23-001, 2023.

[57] HHS, ACF, "HHS Announces New Efforts to Improve Teen Pregnancy Prevention & Sexual Risk Avoidance Programs," press release, November 3, 2017, https://www.acf.hhs.gov/archive/media/press/2017/hhs-announces-new-efforts-improve-teen-pregnancy-prevention-sexual-risk. MITRE's work using these TPP program funds was to occur under the Health FFRDC.

[58] SMARTool was developed by the Center for Relationship Education, a nonprofit organization, with support from the CDC. SMARTool is a program guide for use by schools and other entities that provide sexual risk avoidance education, and it identifies nine protective factors that help prevent sexual risk behaviors in youth. TAC is a resource for use by schools and other entities that describes 17 elements of effective sexual risk reduction programs, which can include sexual risk avoidance approaches or broader approaches such as the use of contraceptives. The tool was developed by ETR Associates and the Healthy Teen Network (nonprofit organizations) with support from the CDC. David Kirby, Lori A. Rolleri, and Mary Martha Wilson, *Tool to Assess the Characteristics of Effective Sex and STD/HIV Education Programs,* ETR and Health Teen Network, 2007.

[59] These activities are described further at USASpending.gov, "Contract Summary, HHS, The MITRE Corporation," https://www.usaspending.gov/#/award/23605015.

(Innovation Networks) grantees for FY2020 and FY2021 implemented each grant strategy and develop recommendations for additional TPP evaluation options. The contract period for this evaluation was September 2021 through April 2024.[60]

HHS-led TPP research and evaluation projects that are currently underway include the following:[61]

- Teenage Pregnancy Prevention Evaluation and Research Grants (Performance Period: September 30, 2022-September 29, 2024). Four grantees will "explore new questions in teen pregnancy prevention, adolescent sexual and reproductive health, and family planning more broadly that improve the efficiency, effectiveness, and quality of these programs for adolescents or young adults, and/or reduce existing disparities."[62]
- Research to Practice Center Grants (Performance Period: September 30, 2022- September 29, 2026). Two grantees will "synthesize and translate existing research into practice for health promotion activities that will lead to adoption of healthy behaviors, improve adolescent health more broadly, and ultimately help to reduce teen pregnancy."[63]

Reproductive Health National Training Center

In 2020, HHS OPA and Office on Women's Health (OWH) awarded a set of three cooperative agreements to JSI Research & Training Institute, Inc. (JSI) to establish and operate a National Training Center for Family Planning and Teen Pregnancy Prevention.[64] Named the Reproductive Health National Training Center (RHNTC), its purpose is to "ensure that personnel working in

---

[60] HHS, OASH, OPA, *Teen Pregnancy Prevention Tier 1 and 2 Evaluation Overview,* https://opa.hhs.gov/sites/default/files/2022-04/tpp-fy2020-fy2021-evaluation-overview_0.pdf.

[61] For further detail on the work to be conducted by each grantee, as well as other ongoing program evaluations, see OASH, OPA, "Current TPP Research & Evaluation Grantees," https://opa.hhs.gov/research-evaluation/teen-pregnancy-prevention-program-evaluations/current-tpp-research-evaluation-grantees.

[62] These grantees are AMTC & Associates; State University of New Jersey, Rutgers; University of Maryland, Baltimore; and University of South Florida.

[63] These grantees are Child Trends, Inc.; and Healthy Teen Network.

[64] According to the FOA, a maximum of $7.4 million would be available for the first 12-month budget period of a project not to exceed five years between the three cooperative agreements funded by Title X, TPP, and OWH. (See HHS, OASH, OPA, and Office of Women's Health (OWH) FOA, "National Training Center for Family Planning and Teen Pregnancy Prevention, PA-FPT-20-001 / AH-TPS-20-001 / WH-AST-20-002, p. 4.)

OPA-funded Title X[65] and TPP projects have the knowledge, skills, and attitudes necessary to deliver high-quality services and programs."[66] The RHNTC allows users to filter through resources by specific program (i.e., TPP or Title X) and includes resources on topics ranging from youth-friendly care and the promotion of healthy relationships to strategies for improved clinic efficiency and quality.[67]

Personal Responsibility Education Program (PREP)

The Personal Responsibility Education Program (PREP) seeks to educate adolescents ages 10 through 19, and pregnant and parenting youth under age 21, on both abstinence and contraceptives to prevent pregnancy and STIs.[68] The Patient Protection and Affordable Care Act (ACA, P.L. 111-148) established PREP by amending Title V of the Social Security Act (SSA) and appropriating $75 million annually in mandatory spending for FY2010 through FY2014.[69] PREP authorization and funding has been extended multiple times, most recently through December 31, 2024, under Division G of the Consolidated Appropriations Act, 2024 (CAA 2024, P.L. 118-42).

PREP funds states and other entities to carry out sexual education programs that place "substantial emphasis on both abstinence and contraception." Recipients of PREP funds must fulfill requirements outlined in the law, including that they must implement programs that

- provide youth with information on at least three of six specified adulthood preparation subjects (healthy relationships, adolescent development, financial literacy, parent-child communication, educational and career success, and healthy life skills);
- are "medically-accurate and complete";

[65] For further information about Title X, see CRS In Focus IF10051, *Title X Family Planning Program*.

[66] See https://rhntc.org/about.

[67] Ibid.

[68] The Personal Responsibility Education Program acronym "PREP" is similar to "PrEP," which refers to pre-exposure prophylaxis medication, which is used to reduce the risk of HIV infection. This report uses PREP to exclusively refer to the adolescent pregnancy prevention programs, although some programs may focus on STI prevention. This report does not cover other federal programs focused on HIV prevention or treatment.

[69] Section 513 of the Social Security Act (42 U.S.C. §513).

- include activities to educate youth who are sexually active regarding responsible sexual behavior with respect to both abstinence and the use of contraception; and
- provide age-appropriate information and activities, while ensuring these are delivered in the most appropriate cultural context for the individuals served in the program.[70]

As with the TPP program, PREP uses a tiered-evidence approach. Nearly all participants in programs implemented by PREP grantees are evidence-based and been proven to delay sexual activity, increase condom or contraceptive use for sexually active youth, or reduce pregnancy among youth.[71] Other grantees substantially incorporate elements of effective programs that have been proven to change behavior. As specified in the law, grantees must serve youth who are ages 10 through 19 and are the most high-risk or vulnerable for pregnancies or otherwise have special circumstances, including youth who are in foster care, are homeless, live with HIV/AIDS, or reside in areas with high birth rates for youth. The program can also serve pregnant youth or mothers under age 21.

PREP includes four types of grants: (1) State PREP grants, (2) Competitive PREP grants, (3) Tribal PREP, and (4) Personal Responsibility Education Innovative Strategies (PREIS). Most of the PREP appropriation is allocated to states and insular areas (Puerto Rico, the U.S. Virgin Islands, Guam, American Samoa, the Commonwealth of the Northern Mariana Islands, the Federated States of Micronesia, the Republic of the Marshall Islands, and the Republic of Palau) via the State PREP grant. Funding for states and insular areas that did not apply for this grant is available to local entities under Competitive PREP grants. The law specifies certain levels of funding for the other components, including $10 million for the PREIS grants. After this set-

[70] The law defines "medically accurate and complete" as verified or supported by research that is conducted in compliance with accepted scientific methods *and* published in peer-reviewed journals, where applicable, or comprising information that leading professional organizations and agencies with relevant expertise in the field recognize as accurate, objective, and complete. This definition is generally consistent with the definition of "medically accurate" used in the other three programs. The law defines "age-appropriate" as topics, messages, and teaching methods that are suitable to particular ages of children and adolescents, based on their developing cognitive, emotional, and behavioral capacity.

[71] HHS, ACF, *FY2025 Justification of Estimates for Appropriations Committee*, p. 266. A review of PREP grantees and participants in 2013 and 2014 found that more than 95% of youth were in programs with evidence-based models. See HHS, OPRE and FYSB, *Personal Responsibility Education Program: A Snapshot of the PREP Performance Measures Report to Congress*, July 2015.

aside, HHS must reserve 5% for grants to Indian tribes and tribal organizations (Tribal PREP) and 10% for training, technical assistance, and evaluation. Total FY2024 funding for the four grants was $75.0 million. Of this amount, $42.8 million was allocated for State PREP, $12.4 million was for Competitive PREP, $3.3 million was for Tribal PREP, and $10.7 million was for PREIS.[72]

State PREP and Competitive PREP

The 50 states, District of Columbia, and insular areas are eligible for State PREP funding. Funds are allocated by a formula that is based on the proportion of youth ages 10 through 19 in each jurisdiction relative to other jurisdictions. State PREP funds do not require a match. A total of 51 jurisdictions applied for and received FY2022 PREP funding for the period of October 1, 2021, through September 30, 2024. This included 44 states, plus the District of Columbia, Guam, the Northern Mariana Islands, Puerto Rico, the Republic of Palau, the Virgin Islands, and the Federated States of Micronesia.[73] States and insular areas can administer the project directly or through sub-awards to public or private entities.

If a state or insular area did not submit an application for formula funding for FY2010 or FY2011, it is ineligible to apply for that formula funding through December 31, 2024.[74]

Organizations in such a state or insular area are eligible to apply competitively for funding, which is to be awarded as a three-year grant. In practice, Competitive PREP applicants can include county or city governments, public institutions of higher education, and for-profit and

---

[72] Ibid.

[73] See *Table B-1* for a list of states receiving the formula grant (from HHS, ACF, FYSB, *State Personal Responsibility Education Program (PREP) Grantees FY2022,* December 31, 2022, https://www.acf.hhs.gov/fysb/grant-funding/state- personal-responsibility-education-program-prep-grantees.) Guam did not apply for State PREP funding for FY2010 through FY2015, and funding instead was awarded under Competitive PREP. Guam first received State PREP funds for FY2016. Similarly, the Northern Mariana Islands did not apply for State PREP funding for FY2010 through FY2016, and funding was provided under Competitive PREP. The Northern Mariana Islands first received State PREP funds for FY2017. (Based on CRS correspondence with HHS, December 2019.)

[74] The law originally stated that jurisdictions that did not submit an application in FY2010 or FY2011 were ineligible to apply for funding in FY2010 through FY2014. Amendments to the law shifted the latter years to FY2015 (P.L. 113- 93), FY2017 (P.L. 114-10), FY2019 (P.L. 115-123), November 21, 2019 (P.L. 116-59), December 20, 2019 (P.L. 116-69), May 22, 2020 (P.L. 116-94), November 30, 2020 (P.L. 116-136), FY2023 (P.L. 116-260), and through December 31, 2024 (P.L. 118-42).

nonprofit organizations, among other entities.[75] HHS awarded Competitive PREP funding for FY2012- FY2014 to organizations located in states that did not apply for funding in FY2010 or FY2011, and awarded a second cohort Competitive PREP funding for FY2015-FY2020.[76] In FY2021, HHS awarded a third cohort of Competitive PREP funds for FY2021 to 27 grantees in Florida, Indiana, Kansas, North Dakota, Texas, and Virginia.[77] HHS noncompetitively continued PREP funding for FY2022 and FY2023, and issued a notice of funding opportunity for FY2024 funds, due June 24, 2024.[78]

Each State PREP and Competitive PREP applicant must include a description of its plan for using the allotment to achieve its goals related to reducing pregnancy rates and birth rates for youth populations.[79] Applicants are required to specify the populations they will serve, and such populations must be the most high-risk or vulnerable for pregnancies or otherwise have special circumstances. States, insular areas, and entities that apply for State

[75] HHS, ACF, FYSB, *FY 2024 Competitive Personal Responsibility Education Program (PREP),* HHS-2024-ACF- ACYF-AK-0032, 2024.

[76] The length of this grant period was related, in part, to a series of short-term funding extensions for PREP that were enacted during this period. The Bipartisan Budget Act of 2018 (BBA 2018, P.L. 115-123) extended the funding period for the grantees through FY2019. As a result, HHS did not publish funding announcements for FY2018 or FY2019 for Competitive PREP or any other component of PREP. (Based on CRS correspondence with HHS, December 2019.) Funding was subsequently extended, most recently through FY2023 (CAA 2021, P.L. 116-260). The FY2022 budget request noted that the project period for 20 of the 21 Competitive PREP grantees was FY2015 through FY2020, with the remaining grantee being extended through January 2022. HHS, ACF, *FY 2022 Justification of Estimates for Appropriations Committee*, p. 286.

[77] HHS, ACF, FYSB, "Competitive Personal Responsibility Education Program (PREP) Grantees FY2021," October 7, 2021, https://www.acf.hhs.gov/fysb/grant-funding/fysb/competitive-personal-responsibility-education-program-prep- grantees-fy2021.

[78] See *Table B-1* for a list of the states with competitive grantees (from HHS, ACF, FYSB, "Competitive Personal Responsibility Education Program (PREP) Grantees FY2023," February 5, 2024, https://www.acf.hhs.gov/fysb/grant- funding/fysb/competitive-personal-responsibility-education-program-prep-grantees.) See also HHS, ACF, FYSB, *FY 2024 Competitive Personal Responsibility Education Program (PREP),* HHS-2024-ACF-ACYF-AK-0032, 2024. Note that although New Hampshire applied for State PREP funding in FY2021 and FY2022, it opted to discontinue receiving State PREP funds for FY2023. As a consequence, entities within New Hampshire were eligible to apply for competitive funds for FY2023; such funds were awarded to two New Hampshire organizations. Eligible FY2024 competitive PREP applicants are limited to local organizations and entities or consortia in the following states and insular areas: Florida, Idaho, Indiana, Kansas, New Hampshire, North Dakota, Texas, Virginia, American Samoa, and the Marshall Islands.

[79] HHS, ACF, FYSB, *State Personal Responsibility Education Program (PREP), Funding Opportunity Announcement and Instructions (for FY2016 and FY2017),* HHS-2016-ACF-ACYF-PREP-1138, 2016; and HHS, ACF, FYSB, *FY 2024 Competitive Personal Responsibility Education Program (PREP),* HHS-2024-ACF-ACYF-AK-0032, 2024.

PREP or Competitive PREP funds must replicate evidence-based adolescent pregnancy prevention programs or substantially incorporate elements of effective programs.[80]

Grantee Profile: Massachusetts

The PREP program in Massachusetts serves youth ages 10 through 19 and pregnant or parenting youth up to age 21. Providers focus on populations with the greatest disparities in reproductive health outcomes in the state, including Hispanic and Latino youth, African-American youth, gender and sexual minority youth, youth in or aging out of foster care, youth with physical and intellectual disabilities, and pregnant or parenting youth. The program implements the following evidence-based curricula in school and community-based settings: It Pays: Partners for Youth Success, Making Proud Choices!, Teen Outreach Program, Be Proud! Be Responsible!, and Get Real. The program also educates its youth in three of the adulthood preparation subjects: adolescent development, financial literacy, and healthy relationships.

Source: HHS, Administration for Children and Families (ACF), Family and Youth Services Bureau (FYSB), State Personal Responsibility Education Program (PREP) Grantee Profiles, August 24, 2017.

Note: This report includes examples of grantees recently funded under the four teen pregnancy prevention programs. The grantees were selected by CRS based on information available on the HHS website or provided via correspondence with HHS. Collectively, the grantees described in the report are intended to represent all regions of the country and are included for illustrative purposes only.

Tribal PREP

Tribal PREP competitive grants are intended to support projects that educate American Indian and Alaska Native youth ages 10 to 20 and pregnant and parenting youth under age 21 on abstinence and contraception for the prevention of pregnancy, STIs, and HIV/AIDS. Specifically, grantees must support the design, implementation, and sustainability of culturally and

[80] Grantees are referred to the Teen Pregnancy Prevention Evidence Review, though they are not required to adopt the models identified in the review.

linguistically appropriate adolescent pregnancy programs. Such programs must replicate evidence-based models, sustainably incorporate elements of effective models, or include promising practices within tribal communities.[81] Indian tribes and tribal organizations, as these terms are defined in the Indian Health Care Improvement Act (P.L. 94-437; 25 U.S.C. §1601), are eligible to apply for Tribal PREP funding. The first cohort of 15 grantees received funding from FY2011 through FY2015.[82] The second cohort of eight grantees received funding from FY2016 through FY2020.[83] The project period for the third cohort of eight grantees (in seven states) that was awarded in FY2021 is five years.[84]

Personal Responsibility Education Innovative Strategies (PREIS)

PREIS competitive grants are intended to build evidence for promising adolescent pregnancy prevention programs serving high-risk youth populations. The grants are awarded on a competitive basis to public and private entities to implement and evaluate innovative youth pregnancy prevention strategies that have not been rigorously evaluated and/or to participate in a federal evaluation of their program strategies if selected.

According to the most recent program funding announcement, innovative strategies could include those that are technology-based and/or computer-based, use social media, or are implemented in nontraditional classroom settings. Such strategies must be targeted to high-risk, vulnerable, and culturally under-represented youth populations.[85] The law specifies that this includes youth ages 10 to 20 in or aging out of foster care; homeless youth; youth with HIV/AIDS; pregnant and parenting women who are under age 21 and their partners; young people residing in areas with high birth rates for

---

[81] HHS, ACF, FYSB, Tribal Personal Responsibility Education Program for Teen Pregnancy Prevention, HHS-2021- ACF-ACYF-AT-1922, 2021.

[82] HHS, ACF, FYSB, 2015 Tribal Personal Responsibility Education Grant Awards, https://www.acf.hhs.gov/fysb/ resource/2015-tribal-prep.

[83] HHS, ACF, FYSB, *Tribal Personal Responsibility Program (PREP) Awards FY2017*, https://www.acf.hhs.gov/fysb/ tribal-prep-awards-fy2017. See also HHS, ACF, *FY 2021 Justification of Estimates for Appropriations Committee*, p. 281.

[84] HHS, ACF, FYSB, *Tribal Personal Responsibility Education Program (PREP) Grantees FY2021,* December 30, 2022, https://www.acf.hhs.gov/fysb/grant-funding/tribal-personal-responsibility-education-program-prep-grantees. One grantee, Tewa Women United, was not continued after FY2021.

[85] HHS, ACF, FYSB, *Personal Responsibility Education Program Innovative Strategies (PREIS)*, HHS-2021-ACF- ACYF-AP-1928, 2021.

youth; and victims of human trafficking. HHS also lists other selected youth populations in the program funding announcement: youth who have been trafficked, runaway and homeless youth, and rural youth.[86] PREIS funds are awarded as five-year cooperative agreements. The first cohort of PREIS grantees, funded for FY2011 through FY2015, included 11 organizations.[87] The second cohort of grantees, funded for FY2016 through FY2020, included 13 organizations in 10 states plus the District of Columbia.[88] The third cohort of grantees, funded in FY2021 with a five-year project period, included 12 organizations in nine states plus the District of Columbia.[89]

PREP Evaluation Activities

PREP authorizing law directs HHS to evaluate PREP programs and activities.[90] The *PREP Multi- Component Evaluation* (2011-2021) supported the first cohort of PREP grantees. The activities of this evaluation included (1) describing how states have designed and implemented PREP programs, (2) collecting and analyzing performance measurement data, and (3) conducting a random assignment evaluation of grantees that receive State PREP or Competitive PREP funding.[91] The study of the grantees overall found that the largest share of youth served by PREP programs have been ages 13 through 16, and over one quarter of programs served the most highly vulnerable youth (e.g., those who were in foster care, identified as LGBTQ, were in residential treatment for mental health issues).[92] Further, youth tended to be served primarily through schools, during school hours. About three quarters of the

---

[86] Ibid.

[87] HHS, ACF, FYSB, *2015 Personal Responsibility Education Innovative Strategies (PREIS) Grant Awards*, https://www.acf.hhs.gov/fysb/resource/2015-preis.

[88] HHS, ACF, FYSB, *Personal Responsibility Education Innovative Strategies (PREIS) Program Awards FY2017*, https://www.acf.hhs.gov/fysb/preis-awards-fy2017; and HHS, ACF, *FY 2022 Justification of Estimates for Appropriations Committee*, p. 286.

[89] HHS, ACF, FYSB, *Personal Responsibility Education Innovative Strategies (PREIS) Program Grantees FY2021*, October 6, 2021, https://www.acf.hhs.gov/fysb/grant-funding/fysb/personal-responsibility-education-innovative- strategies-preis-program.

[90] Section 513(c)(2(B)(iii) of the Social Security Act.

[91] HHS, ACF, OPRE, *Personal Responsibility Education Program (PREP) Multi-Component Evaluation*, https://www.acf.hhs.gov/opre/project/personal-responsibility-education-prog ram-prep-multi-component-evaluation- 2011-2021.

[92] HHS, ACF, Office of Policy Research and Evaluation (OPRE), *Personal Responsibility Education Program (PREP) Evaluation: Nationwide Implementation of PREP Programs*, OPRE Report Number 2018-23, April 2018; HHS, ACF, OPRE, *Inputs and Outcomes: PREP Programs Serving Highly Vulnerable Youth*, OPRE Report #2018-45, April 2018.

youth reported that participating in PREP made them more prepared for adulthood.[93]

The *PREP Studies of Performance Measures and Adulthood Preparation Subjects* (2016-2024) supported the second cohort of PREP grantees. This evaluation was comprised of two key components related to performance measures for PREP and adulthood preparation subjects (APS). The multiple purposes of this project included revising measures used for PREP grantee reporting of performance data, creating a performance dashboard tool, and developing APS conceptual models.[94] In addition, grantee training technical support for the second cohort was provided via the *Promising Youth Programs Project*.[95]

Grantee Profile: Kentucky Department of Health

The Reducing the Risk teen pregnancy prevention curriculum is designed to help teens prevent pregnancy and the transmission of STIs by developing skills such as risk assessment, communication, decisionmaking, planning, and refusal strategies. The Kentucky Department of Health tested the efficacy of providing the curriculum over a shorter duration (8 hours instead of 12 hours) for students in a rural area of the state. The treatment group enrolled in Reducing the Risk (which still covered the same topics, just in a shorter period) and the control group received the school's standard health curriculum. The adapted version reduced the likelihood of having sex without a condom among students who were already sexually active, but it did not change the likelihood of having sex or having sex without a condom for the overall sample.

Source: HHS, ACF, OPRE, Personal Responsibility Education Program (PREP) Evaluation: Evaluating a Teen Pregnancy Prevention Program in Rural Kentucky, OPRE Report Number 2018-105, October 2018.

---

[93] HHS, ACF, OPRE, PREP Studies of Performance Measures and Adult Preparation Subjects, Fact Sheet, 2020-2021 Performance Measures, OPRE Report #2023-029, February 2023.

[94] ACF, ACF, OPRE, *Personal Responsibility Education Program (PREP) Studies of Performance Measures and Adulthood Preparation Subjects,* https://www.acf.hhs.gov/opre/project/prep-studies-performance-measures-and-adulthood-preparation-subjects-2016-2022.

[95] ACF, ACF, OPRE, *Promising Youth Programs Project*, https://www.acf.hhs.gov/fysb/programs/adolescent-pregnancy-prevention/evaluation/promising-youth-programs-project.

Note: This report includes examples of grantees recently funded under the four teen pregnancy prevention programs. The grantees were selected by CRS based on information available on the HHS website or provided via correspondence with HHS. Collectively, the grantees described in the report are intended to represent all regions of the country and are included for illustrative purposes only.

Currently, the *PREP Local Evaluation Support and Dissemination (PLESD)* project provides support for grantees to conduct rigorous program evaluations and to build research and evaluation capacity. This support for grantees is expected to extend through 2026.[96]

Separate from these evaluation efforts, PREIS and Tribal PREP grantees are directed to carry out evaluation activities. PREIS grantees must contract with independent third-party evaluators to conduct RCT or quasi-experimental research to determine whether grantees' interventions led to outcomes such as reduced pregnancies, births, and STIs. Tribal PREP grantees must partner with a university or other organization not associated with the grantee to conduct an evaluation (known as a "local evaluation") that is either descriptive (without treatment and comparison groups) or examines impacts using treatment and comparison groups. State PREP and Competitive PREP grantees may choose to conduct such local evaluations.

Title V Sexual Risk Avoidance Education Program (Title V SRAE)

A Separate Program for Abstinence Education was established under Section 510 in Title V of the Social Security Act by The Personal Responsibility and Work Opportunity Reconciliation Act of 1996 (PRWORA, P.L. 104-193). Now named the Title V Sexual Risk Avoidance Education program (Title V SRAE), it is funded through mandatory appropriations in the Social Security Act. When the program was initially established, PRWORA provided $50 million per year for five years (FY1998-FY2002). The program was subsequently funded through June 30, 2009, by various legislative extensions.

[96] ABT Associates, *Personal Responsibility Education Program (PREP) Local Evaluation Support and Dissemination (PLESD)*, https://www.abtassociates.com/projects/providing-local-evaluation-support-to-acfs-prep-grantees.

The ACA reauthorized the program, providing $50 million for each of FY2010 through FY2014.

Title V Sexual Risk Avoidance Education Topics

Sexual risk avoidance education, also sometimes referred to as abstinence-only education, must ensure that the "unambiguous and primary emphasis and context" for each of six sexual risk avoidance topics is "a message to youth that normalizes the optimal health behavior of avoiding nonmarital sexual activity." The sexual risk avoidance topics include the following:

- The holistic individual and societal benefits associated with personal responsibility, self- regulation, goal setting, healthy decisionmaking, and a focus on the future.
- The advantage of refraining from nonmarital sexual activity in order to improve the future prospects and physical and emotional health of youth.
- The increased likelihood of avoiding poverty when youth attain self-sufficiency and emotional maturity before engaging in sexual activity.
- The foundational components of healthy relationships and their impact on the formation of healthy marriages and safe and stable families.
- How other youth risk behaviors, such as drug and alcohol usage, increase the risk for teen sex.
- How to resist, avoid, and receive help regarding sexual coercion and dating violence, recognizing that, even with consent, teen sex remains a youth risk behavior.

Source: Section 510(b)(3) of the Social Security Act.

Multiple subsequent laws extended the program and increased its funding. The Protecting Access to Medicare Act of 2014 (P.L. 113-93) provided $50 million in FY2015. Next, the Medicare Access and CHIP Reauthorization Act of 2015 (P.L. 114-10) increased funding to $75 million per year for FY2016 and FY2017. Two additional fiscal years (FY2018 and FY2019) of funding were enacted by the Bipartisan Budget Act of 2018 (P.L. 115-123, BBA 2018).

Following several temporary extensions, funding has been most recently provided through December 31, 2024, under Division G of the CAA 2024 (P.L. 118-42).

States are eligible to request mandatory Title V SRAE funds if they submit an application for Title V State Maternal and Child Health (MCH) Block Grant funds. The State MCH Block Grant program, authorized under Title V of the Social Security Act, is a flexible source of funds administered through a federal-state partnership which supports a range of maternal and child health programs.[97] Title V SRAE funds are allocated to each jurisdiction based on two factors: (1) the total amount of annual funding provided to the Title V SRAE program in Section 510 minus any reservations (up to 20%) made by HHS for administering it, and (2) states' relative proportion of low-income children nationally.[98] The law does not require states to provide a match.[99]

HHS is authorized to competitively award FY2018 through FY2025 funds to one or more entities within a state/insular area that had not previously applied for its share of funding. (The law does not define the entities that would be eligible.) The HHS Secretary is required to publish a notice to solicit grant applications for any remaining competitive funds. The solicitation must be published within 30 days after the deadline for states to apply for State MCH Block Grant funds. Eligible states are required to apply for the Title V SRAE funds no later than 120 days after the deadline closed for states to apply

---

[97] For further information, see CRS Report R48088, *Maternal and Child Health Services Block Grant: Overview and Issues for Congress*. All states, the District of Columbia, and five insular areas (American Samoa, Guam, the Northern Mariana Islands, Puerto Rico, and the U.S. Virgin Islands), and three freely associated states (Federated States of Micronesia, Republic of the Marshall Islands, and Republic of Palau) receive MCH Block Grant funds. (See HHS, HRSA, Explore the Title V Federal-State Partnership, https://mchb.tvisdata.hrsa.gov/.)

[98] Census data are not available for the Federated States of Micronesia, the Republic of the Marshall Islands, and the Republic of Palau. Thus, the allocations for these three entities, when applicable, are based on the amounts allocated to them by HHS in prior fiscal years. HHS, ACF, FYSB, *Standing Notice of Funding Opportunity for Title V State Sexual Risk Avoidance Education*, HHS-2024-ACF-ACYF-SRAE-0044, 2024.

[99] Previously, such a matching requirement was specified at Section 510(c) of the Social Security Act, which referenced the Maternal and Child Health Block Grant at Section 503. Section 503(a) states that HHS is to fund four- sevenths (approximately 57%) of the program activities under the MCH Services Block Grant. To receive federal funding, a state must match every $4 in federal funds with $3 in state funds—via state dollars, local government dollars, private dollars, or in-kind support—that will be used solely for activities specified in the law. This match applied to the Title V Abstinence Education program. This requirement, as it temporarily applied to the Title V Sexual Risk Avoidance Education program, was struck by the Consolidated Appropriations Act, 2018 (P.L. 115-141).

for State MCH Block Grant funds. The entity or entities would receive the amount that would have been otherwise allotted to that state.

The 50 states, the District of Columbia, and the insular areas (Puerto Rico, U.S. Virgin Islands, Guam, American Samoa, Commonwealth of the Northern Mariana Islands, Federated States of Micronesia, the Republic of the Marshall Islands, and Republic of Palau) are eligible to apply for funding. In total, 36 states plus Puerto Rico and the Federated States of Micronesia applied for and received funding for FY2022-FY2024.[100] Another 34 grantees in 12 states plus Guam and the U.S. Virgin Islands received new Competitive SRAE funding for FY2023-FY2024.[101]

The law directs states/insular areas or other entities to implement sexual risk avoidance education that is medically accurate and complete, age-appropriate, and based on adolescent learning and developmental theories for the age group receiving the education.[102] As described in the previous text box, sexual risk avoidance education must address six topics. According to the grant announcements for the program, if sexual risk avoidance education includes any information about contraception, such information must be medically accurate and ensure that students understand that contraception reduces physical risk but does not eliminate risk. In addition, sexual risk avoidance education may not include demonstration, simulation, or distribution of contraception.

Additionally, the grant announcements have previously specified that grantees must implement a project with a "best practice and/or evidence-based approach." The grant announcements have directed applicants to research documents, such as SMARTool and the CDC's HECAT (Health Education Curriculum Assessment Tool), that identify "critical elements to success in

---

[100] See *Table B-1* for a list of states receiving the formula grant (from HHS, ACF, FYSB, *Title V State Sexual Risk Avoidance Education (SRAE) Grantees FY2022,* https://www.acf.hhs.gov/fysb/grant-funding/fysb/title-v-state-sexual-risk-avoidance-education-srae-grantees).

[101] See *Table B-1* for a list of the states with competitive grantees (from HHS, ACF, FYSB, *Title V Competitive Sexual Risk Avoidance Education (SRAE) Grantees, FY2023,* https://www.acf.hhs.gov/fysb/grant-funding/title-v-competitive-sexual-risk-avoidance-education-srae-grantees).

[102] The law defines "medically accurate and complete" as information verified or supported by research that is conducted in compliance with accepted scientific methods *and* published in peer-reviewed journals, where applicable, or information that leading professional organizations and agencies with relevant expertise in the field recognize as accurate, objective, and complete. This definition is generally consistent with the definition of "medically accurate" used in the other three programs. The law defines "age appropriate" as topics, messages, and teaching methods that are suitable to particular ages of children and adolescents, based their on developing cognitive, emotional, and behavioral capacity.

implementing programs to positively change youth behavior."[103] (For further information, see the "TPP Evaluation Activities" section.) These announcements also have pointed to the TPPER website for a list of evidence-based programs, although applications are not required to implement these approaches.[104]

Title V SRAE Evaluation Activities

Under the authorizing statute, a state or other entity that receives Title V SRAE funding must, as specified by the HHS Secretary, collect information on the programs and activities funded through their allotments and submit reports to HHS on the data collected from such programs and activities. Recent grant announcements for the program have specified that jurisdictions must assess the success of their sexual risk avoidance education programs through at least two outcome measures.[105] Furthermore, a state or other entity receiving funding under the Title V SRAE program may use up to 20% of its allotment to build the evidence base for sexual risk avoidance education by conducting or supporting research. Any such research must be rigorous, evidence- based, and designed and conducted by independent researchers who have experience in conducting and publishing research in peer-reviewed outlets.[106]

Grantee Profile: Arizona

The Title V Abstinence Education program in Arizona is implementing the following education models: Choosing the Best, Love Notes SRA Edition, Making a Difference, Promoting Health Among Teens (PHAT)! Abstinence Only, and the Teen Outreach Program (TOP). The target population is youth ages 11 through 19 who are in areas across the state

[103] See, for example, *Standing Announcement for Title V State Sexual Risk Avoidance Education*, HHS-2020-ACF- ACYF-SRAE-1848, 2020.

[104] See, for example, HHS, ACF, FYSB, *Title V Competitive Sexual Risk Avoidance Education (SRAE)*, HHS-2024- ACF-ACYF-SRAE-0040, 2024.

[105] See, for example, HHS, ACF, FYSB, *Standing Notice of Funding Opportunity for Title V State Sexual Risk Avoidance Education*, HHS-2024-ACF-ACYF-SRAE-0044, 2024.

[106] The law defines "rigorous," with respect to research and evaluation, to mean using (1) established scientific methods for ensuring the impact of an intervention or program model in changing behavior (specifically sexual activity or other risk behaviors), or reducing pregnancy among youth; or (2) other evidence-based methodologies established by the HHS Secretary for purposes of the Title V Sexual Risk Avoidance Education program.

with high teen pregnancy rates; Hispanic, black, or American Indian youth; and youth in foster care. The program's services are provided by one county health department and with community-based organizations in schools and community-based settings. Generally, the program focuses on the benefits of protective factors to support adolescents' decisions in refraining from nonmarital sex, including healthy relationships, setting goals, self- regulation, and academic success. In addition to the curriculum above, the program may deliver an optional parental education component to parents of youth aged 11 through 19.

Sources: HHS, ACF, FYSB, Title V State Sexual Risk Avoidance Education (SRAE) Grantee Profiles, April 2, 2021; and Arizona Department of Health Services, Title V State Sexual Risk Avoidance Education Program State Plan, 2018.

Note: In the absence of information about Title V Sexual Risk Avoidance Education grantees on the HHS website, this grantee was selected by CRS based on an internet search. Collectively, the grantees described in the report are intended to represent all regions of the country and are included for illustrative purposes only.

Separately, the law as amended by the BBA 2018, requires HHS to conduct one or more rigorous evaluations of the education (and associated data) funded through the Title V SRAE program.

This evaluation is to be conducted in consultation with "appropriate State and local agencies." HHS is to also consult with relevant stakeholders and evaluation experts about the evaluation(s). HHS must submit a report to Congress on the results of the evaluation(s). The report must also include a summary of the information collected and reported by states and other entities on their Title V SRAE programs and activities.

HHS has contracted with Mathematica Policy Research, in partnership with Public Strategies, to conduct evaluation activities under what is known as the Sexual Risk Avoidance National Evaluation (SRANE). The evaluation is a five-year study that includes both Title V SRAE grantees and SRAE program grantees funded under the General Departmental Management account (see the "General Department Sexual Risk Avoidance Education Program (GD SRAE)" section for further information), and has three components:

1) National Descriptive Study: This will describe SRAE grantees' program plans (Early Implementation Study) and examine grantees' implementation and youth outcomes (Nationwide Study).
2) Program Components Impacts Study: This will provide an analysis of promising program approaches and the effectiveness of SRAE program components (e.g., parent engagement and/or staff training strategies). It will not evaluate the effectiveness of the full program.
3) Data Capacity Building and Local Evaluation Support: This component focuses on supporting grantees in collecting and using local data to improve their programs and support grantee-funded evaluations.[107]

In addition, the *Sexual Risk Avoidance Education Performance Analysis Study* (2019-2027) is intended to collect performance measures data from Title V SRAE program participants and providers to allow both the program office and grantees to monitor and report on progress in implementing SRAE initiatives. Primary activities include support to grantees to collect and submit performance measures, the development of a portal for performance measures submission, and development of a dashboard for use by grantees and the program office for continuous quality improvement. The contract for this evaluation was awarded to Public Strategies (with Mathematica as a subcontractor) for FY2019-FY2023, and to Mathematica (with Public Strategies as a subcontractor) for FY2022-FY2027.[108]

With regard to the prior Title V Abstinence Education Grant program, the Balanced Budget Act of 1997 (P.L. 105-133) directed HHS to conduct evaluation activities.[109] In response, HHS undertook a multi-year evaluation that included a study of how grantees in four states implemented abstinence education programs and a separate study that rigorously evaluated whether grantees' programs had impacts on adolescent sexual abstinence and related outcomes.

---

[107] HHS, ACF, OPRE, *Sexual Risk Avoidance Education National Evaluation, 2018 – 2023*, https://www.acf.hhs.gov/ opre/research/project/sexual-risk-avoidance-education-national-evaluation; and HHS, ACF, FYSB and OPRE, *Looking Back, Moving Forward: SRAE National Evaluation Frequently Asked questions,* https://sraene.com/sites/default/files/ pdfs/SRAENE_FAQ.pdf. Several SRANE studies have been published at https://www.acf.hhs.gov/opre/project/sexual-risk-avoidance-education-national-evaluation-2018-2023.

[108] HHS, ACF, OPRE, *Sexual Risk Avoidance Education Performance Analysis Study*, https://www.acf.hhs.gov/opre/project/sexual-risk-avoidance-education-performance-analysis-study-2019-2022.

[109] P.L. 105-133 did not amend Title V of the Social Security Act.

The programs enrolled youth in elementary and middle school and engaged them as part of the school setting, including in afterschool programming. Each individual participated for more than 50 hours. The study tracked longitudinal outcomes among participants for four and six years after they were enrolled in the program. The impact evaluation found that youth who received abstinence education under the program did not have different outcomes than youth in the control in terms of likelihood to abstain from sex, number of sexual partners, and mean age of initiation.[110]

General Department Sexual Risk Avoidance Education Program (GD SRAE)

In the past, federal funding supported abstinence-only education through the Community-Based Abstinence Education program (FY2001 through FY2009) and the Competitive Abstinence-Only program (FY2012 through FY2015). In each of FY2016 through FY2024, annual appropriations laws provided funding to support abstinence-only education through the General Department Sexual Risk Avoidance Education (GD SRAE) program. Funding was $5 million in FY2016, $15 million in FY2017, $25 million in FY2018, and $35 million in FY2019 through FY2024. The appropriations laws have specified that GD SRAE grants are to

- be awarded by HHS on a competitive basis;
- use medically accurate information;
- "implement an evidence-based approach integrating research findings with practical implementation that aligns with the needs and desired outcomes for the intended audience;" and
- "teach the benefits associated with self-regulation, success sequencing for poverty prevention, healthy relationships, goal setting, and resisting sexual coercion, dating violence, and other youth risk behaviors such as underage drinking or illicit drug use without normalizing teen sexual activity."[111]

---

[110] Barbara Devaney, *The Evaluation of Abstinence Education Programs Funded Under Title V Section 510: Interim Report*, Mathematica Policy Research, Inc., for HHS, OPRE, April 2002; and Christopher Trenholm et al., *Impacts of Four Title V, Section 510 Abstinence Education Programs: Final Report*, Mathematica Policy Research, Inc., for HHS, ACF, ASPE, April 2007.

[111] This text has been included in each of the appropriation laws for FY2016 through FY2024.

The appropriations laws have provided that up to 10% of the funding for sexual risk avoidance can be made available for technical assistance and administrative costs.

Through the grant application process for the GD SRAE program, HHS has identified multiple types of entities that are eligible for funding, including states, territories, and localities (county, city, township, special districts); school districts; public and state-controlled institutions of higher education; federally recognized tribal governments; Native American tribal organizations; public and Indian housing authorities; nonprofit organizations other than institutions of higher education; private institutions of higher education; small business; and for-profit organizations other than small businesses.[112] GD SRAE grants are awarded for two-year project periods, typically with some new and some noncompetitive continuations each year. Most recently, HHS awarded 31 new grants for FY2021 (totaling $12.8 million, FY2021-FY2022 project period) and noncompetitively continued 51 grants (totaling $21.5 million, FY2021-FY2022 project period); grants were noncompetitively continued for FY2022 and FY2023.[113] HHS has also issued a notice of funding opportunity for FY2024 funds, due June 24, 2024.[114]

As specified in the funding announcements, grantees must incorporate an evidence-based program and/or effective strategies that have demonstrated impacts on delaying the initiation of sexual activity. HHS advises that grantees provide data that demonstrate how the selected curriculum and their proposals apply key program elements that have been found to be effective in promoting positive youth behavior changes, especially delaying sexual activity, returning to a lifestyle without sex, and refraining from nonmarital sex. The grant announcements point out that such elements have been identified in research summary documents such as HECAT (discussed in the "TPP Evaluation Activities" section), and the TPPER, but applicants are not required to implement these approaches.[115]

---

[112] HHS, ACF, FYSB, General Departmental Sexual Risk Avoidance Education (GD-SRAE), HHS-2024-ACF-ACYF- SR-0041, 2024.

[113] HHS, ACF, FYSB, *General Departmental Sexual Risk Avoidance Education (GD SRAE) Grantees (FY2021, FY2022, FY2023)*, https://www.acf.hhs.gov/fysb/grant-funding/fysb/general-departmental-sexual-risk-avoidance- education-gd-srae-grantees. See *Table B-1* for a list of states with GD SRAE grantees for FY2023.

[114] HHS, ACF, FYSB, *General Departmental Sexual Risk Avoidance Education (GD-SRAE)*, HHS-2024-ACF-ACYF- SR-0041, 2024.

[115] HHS, ACF, ACYF, *Sexual Risk Avoidance Education Program*, HHS-2021-ACF-ACYF-SR-1927, 2021. HHS, ACF, FYSB, *General Departmental Sexual Risk Avoidance Education (GD-SRAE)*, HHS-2024-ACF-ACYF-SR-0041, 2024.

Grantee Profile: Healthy Visions in Ohio

HHS awarded FY2023-FY2024 Sexual Risk Avoidance Education funding to Healthy Visions, a social services organization located in Cincinnati, OH. The organization implements four curricula: Real Essentials, Choosing the Best, Love Notes, and TYRO Rites of Passage. The program serves youth in grades 4-12 in school-based settings. The curricula focus on topics such as risk avoidance (such as delaying sex), setting goals, healthy relationships, communication skills, conflict resolution, stress management, and self-respect.

Source: HHS, ACF, FYSB, General Departmental Sexual Risk Avoidance Education (SRAE) Program Grantee Profiles, February 11, 2022; and Healthy Visions, "Quick Look," https://healthyvisions.org/quick-look/.

Note: This report includes examples of grantees recently funded under the four teen pregnancy prevention programs. The grantees were selected by CRS based on information available on the HHS website or provided via correspondence with HHS. Collectively, the grantees described in the report are intended to represent all regions of the country and are included for illustrative purposes only.

Appendix A. Federal Teen Pregnancy Prevention Programs

Table A-1. Federal teen pregnancy prevention programs: overview, eligible entities, and funding

Program Feature	Teen Pregnancy Prevention (TPP) Program	Personal Responsibility Education Program	Title V Sexual Risk Avoidance Education Program[a]	GD Sexual Risk Avoidance Education Program
Authorizing law (and statutory citation, where applicable)	Initial authorizing law was the Consolidated Appropriations Act, 2010 (P.L. 111-117) and authority has continued under subsequent appropriation laws. The most recent appropriations law is Division D of the Further Consolidated Appropriations Act, 2024 (P.L. 118-47).	Patient Protection and Affordable Care Act (ACA, P.L. 111-148), most recently reauthorized through December 31, 2024 under Division G of the Consolidated Appropriations Act, 2024 (CAA 2024, P.L. 118-42).	Personal Responsibility and Work Opportunity Reconciliation Act of 1996 (P.L. 104-193), most recently reauthorized through December 31, 2024 under Division G of the CAA 2024 (P.L. 118-42).	Initial authorizing law was the Consolidated Appropriations Act, 2016 (P.L. 114-113) and authority has continued under subsequent appropriation laws. The most recent appropriations law is Division D of the Further Consolidated Appropriations Act, 2024 (P.L. 118-47). HHS additionally cites its general authority to administer the program (42 U.S.C. §1310) in its program funding announcements.[b]

Table A-1. (Continued)

Program Feature	Teen Pregnancy Prevention (TPP) Program	Personal Responsibility Education Program	Title V Sexual Risk Avoidance Education Program[a]	GD Sexual Risk Avoidance Education Program
Description	The program funds grantees to replicate programs that have been proven effective in reducing teen pregnancy and behavioral risk factors underlying teenage pregnancy (Tier 1 grants); and to develop, test, and refine additional programs and strategies for preventing teenage pregnancy (Tier 2 grants).	The program funds states, insular areas, and other entities, under four components: State PREP, Competitive PREP, Tribal PREP, and Personal Responsibility Education Innovative Strategies (PREIS). "Personal responsibility education program" refers to a program that is (1) designed to educate adolescents on both abstinence and contraception for the prevention of pregnancy and sexually transmitted infections (STIs), including HIV/AIDS; and (2) incorporate at least three of six adult preparatory subjects (healthy relationships, adolescent	The program funds states and insular areas (or other entities in a jurisdiction that did not apply for funds) to implement education exclusively on sexual risk avoidance, meaning voluntarily refraining from sexual activity. Sexual risk avoidance education must ensure that the "unambiguous and primary emphasis and context" for each of six sexual risk avoidance topics specified in the law is "a message to youth that normalizes the optimal health behavior of avoiding nonmarital sexual activity." If any information is provided	The program funds grantees to implement sexual risk avoidance education that teaches participants how to voluntarily refrain from nonmarital sexual activity and prevent other youth risk behaviors.

Program Feature	Teen Pregnancy Prevention (TPP) Program	Personal Responsibility Education Program	Title V Sexual Risk Avoidance Education Program[a]	GD Sexual Risk Avoidance Education Program
		development, financial literacy, education and career success, parent-child communication, and healthy life skills)	about contraception, it must be medically accurate and ensure that students understand that contraception reduces physical risk, but does not eliminate risk. In addition, it may not include demonstration, simulation, or distribution of contraception.	
Administering agency within the U.S. Department of Health and Human Services (HHS)	Office of Population Affairs (OPA) within the Office of the Assistant Secretary for Health (OASH).	Family and Youth Services Bureau (FYSB) within the Administration for Children and Families (ACF).	FYSB/ACF	FYSB/ACF
Entities eligible to apply, and how funds are awarded	Eligible entities are specified in the program funding announcements. Eligible entities vary depending on the grant, but generally include nonprofit and for-profit	As specified in the authorizing law, funds are awarded on a formula basis to states and insular areas under the State PREP	As specified in the authorizing law, all states and insular areas that receive State Maternal and Child	Eligible grantees are specified in the program funding announcements. They have included state, territorial, or county governments; city or

Table A-1. (Continued)

Program Feature	Teen Pregnancy Prevention (TPP) Program	Personal Responsibility Education Program	Title V Sexual Risk Avoidance Education Program[a]	GD Sexual Risk Avoidance Education Program
	organizations; small, minority, and women-owned businesses; state and local governments; universities and colleges; community- and faith-based organizations; hospitals; federally recognized or state-recognized American Indian and Alaska Native tribal governments; and other tribal entities (e.g., Alaska Native health corporations). Funds are awarded on a competitive basis.	program. Funds are allocated based on the proportion of children in each state between the ages of 10 and 19, relative to the total number of youth nationally. State PREP funds that would have been allocated to states that did not apply for them are competitively awarded under the Competitive PREP program. As listed in the program funding announcements, entities eligible to apply for the Competitive PREP program and PREIS generally have included state, territorial, or county governments; city or township governments; special district governments; independent,	Health (MCH) block grant funds in FY2018 through FY2025 are eligible to apply. HHS may competitively award FY2018 through FY2025 funds to one or more entities (not defined) within a state/insular area that had not previously applied for its share of funding. The entity or entities would receive the amount that would have been otherwise allotted to that state/insular area.	township governments; special district governments; independent, regional, and local school districts; public and state controlled institutions of higher education; federally recognized Native American tribal governments; public housing authorities/Indian housing authorities; Native American tribal organizations; nonprofit organizations; private institutions of higher education; for-profit organizations other than small businesses; and small businesses. Funds are awarded on a competitive basis.

Program Feature	Teen Pregnancy Prevention (TPP) Program	Personal Responsibility Education Program	Title V Sexual Risk Avoidance Education Program[a]	GD Sexual Risk Avoidance Education Program
		regional, and local school districts; public and state controlled institutions of higher education; federally recognized Native American tribal governments; public housing authorities/Indian housing authorities; Native American tribal organizations; nonprofit organizations; private institutions of higher education. for-profit organizations other than small businesses; local affiliates of national organizations; and small businesses. Also as listed in the program funding announcement, Indian tribes and tribal organizations, as these terms are defined in the Indian Health Care	Allotments are based on two factors: (1) the amount provided to the program minus any reservations (up to 20%) made by HHS for administering it, and (2) states' relative proportion of low-income children nationally.	

Table A-1. (Continued)

Program Feature	Teen Pregnancy Prevention (TPP) Program	Personal Responsibility Education Program	Title V Sexual Risk Avoidance Education Program[a]	GD Sexual Risk Avoidance Education Program
		Improvement Act, are eligible to apply for Tribal PREP funding.		
Type of funding, year(s) of funding, and funding set-asides (where applicable)	Discretionary spending; funded through appropriations law. Funding is provided for FY2024 as of the cover date of this report. Up to 10% of appropriated funds can be used for training and technical assistance, outreach, and other program support. Of the remaining amount, 75% is to be used to replicate programs (Tier 1 grants) and 25% is to be used for developing, testing, and refining additional models (Tier 2 grants).	Mandatory spending; funded through authorizing law. Funding is authorized through December 31, 2024, as of the cover date of this report. The law provides $10 million for the PREIS grants. After this set-aside, HHS must reserve 5% for grants to Indian tribes and tribal organizations (Tribal PREP) and 10% for training, technical assistance, and evaluation. Most of the remaining PREP appropriation is allocated to states and insular areas via State PREP (with a minimum of $250,000 for	Mandatory spending; funded through authorizing law. Funding is authorized through December 31, 2024, as of the cover date of this report.	Discretionary spending; funded through appropriations law. Funding is authorized for FY2024 as of the cover date of this report.

Program Feature	Teen Pregnancy Prevention (TPP) Program	Personal Responsibility Education Program	Title V Sexual Risk Avoidance Education Program[a]	GD Sexual Risk Avoidance Education Program
		each state allotment). Funding for states and insular areas that declined the State PREP grant is available to eligible entities under Competitive PREP.		
Cost sharing	Not applicable.	Not applicable.	Not applicable.	Not applicable.
Enacted federal funding from FY2010-FY2024[c]	FY2010: $110.0 million FY2011: $104.8 million FY2012: $104.8 million FY2013: $98.3 million FY2014: $100.8 million FY2015: $101.0 million FY2016: $101.0 million FY2017: $100.8 million FY2018: $101.0 million	FY2010: $75.0 million FY2011: $75.0 million FY2012: $75.0 million FY2013: $71.2 million FY2014: $69.6 million FY2015: $75.0 million FY2016: $75.0 million FY2017: $69.8 million FY2018: $75.0 million	FY2010: $50.0 million FY2011: $50.0 million FY2012: $50.0 million FY2013: $47.5 million FY2014: $46.4 million FY2015: $50.0 million FY2016: $75.0 million FY2017: $69.8 million FY2018: $75.0 million	FY2010: Not funded FY2011: Not funded FY2012: $5.0 million FY2013: $4.7 million FY2014: $5.0 million FY2015: $5.0 million FY2016: $10.0 million FY2017: $15.0 million FY2018: $25.0 million
	FY2019: $101.0 million FY2020: $101.0 million FY2021: $101.0 million FY2022: $101.0 million FY2023: $101.0 million FY2024: $101.0 million	FY2019: $75.0 million FY2020: $75.0 million FY2021: $75.0 million FY2022: $70.7 million FY2023: $70.7 million FY2024: $75.0 million	FY2019: $75.0 million FY2020: $75.0 million FY2021: $75.0 million FY2022: $70.7 million FY2023: $70.7 million FY2024: $75.0 million	FY2019: $35.0 million FY2020: $35.0 million FY2021: $35.0 million FY2022: $35.0 million FY2023: $35.0 million FY2024: $35.0 million

Table A-1. (Continued)

Program Feature	Teen Pregnancy Prevention (TPP) Program	Personal Responsibility Education Program	Title V Sexual Risk Avoidance Education Program[a]	GD Sexual Risk Avoidance Education Program
Use of evidence-based interventions	Per the FY2024 appropriations law (P.L. 118-47), "75 percent [of funds] shall be for replicating programs that have been proven effective through rigorous evaluation to reduce teenage pregnancy, behavioral risk factors underlying teenage pregnancy, or other associated risk factors, and 25 percent shall be available for research and demonstration grants to develop, replicate, refine, and test additional models and innovative strategies for preventing teenage pregnancy." Previously, Tier 1 applicants have been referred in the	State PREP jurisdictions and Competitive PREP grantees must replicate evidence-based, effective programs or substantially incorporate elements of effective programs that have been proven on the basis of rigorous scientific research to change behavior. The grant announcements have referred applicants to the TPPER for information on such programs, though other models can be implemented that meet the requirement of being rigorously evaluated. The grant announcements have specified that Tribal PREP grantees are to replicate evidence-based effective programs; substantially incorporate	A state/insular area or other entity receiving funding under the Sexual Risk Avoidance Education program may use up to 20% of such allotment to build the evidence base for sexual risk avoidance by conducting or supporting research. Any such research must be rigorous, evidence-based, and designed and conducted by independent researchers who have experience in conducting and publishing research in peer-reviewed outlets. As specified in the most recent funding announcements, grantees	Per the FY2024 appropriations law (P.L. 118-47), grantees must "implement an evidence-based approach integrating research findings with practical implementation that aligns with the needs and desired outcomes for the intended audience." As specified in the funding announcements, grantees must incorporate an evidence-based program and/or effective strategies that have demonstrated impacts on delaying the initiation of sexual activity. HHS advises that grantees provide data that

Program Feature	Teen Pregnancy Prevention (TPP) Program	Personal Responsibility Education Program	Title V Sexual Risk Avoidance Education Program[a]	GD Sexual Risk Avoidance Education Program
	program funding announcement to the Teen Pregnancy Prevention Evidence Review (TPPER) for information on evidence-based models.	elements of effective programs to the extent possible; or include promising practices within the American Indian/Alaska Native (AI/AN) communities. There are no pregnancy prevention programs specifically for AI/AN communities in the TPP Evidence Review. The grant announcements have specified that PREIS grantees are to use innovative strategies, with promising evidence of effectiveness or impact, but which must not have been rigorously evaluated. Therefore, the evidence-based programs identified in the TPPER are not eligible interventions for this specific program.	must incorporate an evidence-based program and/or effective strategies that have demonstrated impacts on delaying the initiation of sexual activity. HHS advises that grantees provide data that demonstrate how the selected curriculum and their proposals apply key program elements that have been found to be effective in promoting positive youth behavior changes, especially delaying sexual activity, returning to a lifestyle without sex, and refraining from nonmarital sex. The grant announcement points out that such elements have been	demonstrates how the selected curriculum and their proposals apply key program elements that have been found to be effective in promoting positive youth behavior changes, especially delaying sexual activity, returning to a lifestyle without sex, and refraining from nonmarital sex. The grant announcement points out that such elements have been identified in research summary documents such as HECAT.[d]

Table A-1. (Continued)

Program Feature	Teen Pregnancy Prevention (TPP) Program	Personal Responsibility Education Program	Title V Sexual Risk Avoidance Education Program[a]	GD Sexual Risk Avoidance Education Program
			identified in research summary documents such as HECAT.[d]	
Target population	The TPP grants generally do not specify a certain target population (either in the authorizing statute or program funding announcement), with the exception of the Tier 2 Innovation Network grants. The Innovation Network grants are to target one of several key priority areas: juvenile justice, foster care/child welfare, caregivers, expectant and parenting youth, youth with disabilities, youth access to and experience with sexual health care, and youth engagement. The	The authorizing statute specifies that jurisdictions and grantees are generally to provide services to youth ages 10 through 19, with a focus on high-risk or vulnerable youth. This includes youth in or aging out of foster care, homeless youth, youth with HIV/AIDS, pregnant and parenting women under 21 years of age and their partners, and young people residing in areas with high birth rates for youth. Tribal PREP grantees must serve American Indian/Alaska Native (AI/AN) youth age 10	Youth ages 10 through 19.	Per the program funding announcement, grantees are to target youth (defined as ages 10- 19) populations that are at risk for nonmarital sexual activity and other risk behaviors. These at-risk populations are not specifically defined.

Program Feature	Teen Pregnancy Prevention (TPP) Program	Personal Responsibility Education Program	Title V Sexual Risk Avoidance Education Program[a]	GD Sexual Risk Avoidance Education Program
	other grants focus on youth in geographic areas with the greatest need (Tier 1) and addressing disparities in teen pregnancy rates using innovative approaches (Tier 2 Rigorous Evaluation).	through 19 or pregnant and parenting women age 21 and under. Per the program funding announcement, Tribal PREP grantees may serve AI/AN youth who have the additional risk factors previously discussed (and other risk factors such as having experienced sex trafficking).		
Number of youth participants (most recent fiscal year data available)	Grantees served 140,935 youth in FY2023.	Grantees served 87,035 youth in FY2022.	Grantees served 240,055 youth in FY2023.	HHS estimates that approximately 54,000 youth participated in FY2019.
Setting for services (selected examples)	Schools Out-of-school programs Clinics Juvenile justice centers Faith-based organizations Out-of-home care (foster care) Runaway/homeless youth centers	Schools (in school or after school) Community-based organizations Foster care settings Juvenile detention centers Clinics Outpatient and residential treatment facilities for youth with social, emotional, or substance abuse disorders Other settings	(Under the prior Title V Abstinence Education Grant program, school was the primary setting) Schools (in school or after school) Mentoring programs School rallies and assemblies	Schools Community-based organizations Foster care organizations Juvenile detention centers Homeless shelters

Sources: Authorizing and appropriation laws (referenced in table); Congressional Research Service (CRS) correspondence with the U.S. Department of Health and Human Services (HHS), Administration for Children and Families (ACF), Office of the Assistant Secretary for Health (OASH), Office of Population Affairs (OPA, formerly Office of Adolescent Health, OAH) December 2019; HHS, *Fiscal Year 2025 Justification of Estimates for Appropriations Committees for General Departmental Management*, p. 91; and HHS, *Fiscal Year 2025 Justification of Estimates for Appropriations Committee for Administration for Children and Families,* pp. 272-273; and as referenced below.

Teen Pregnancy Prevention (TPP) Program: (1) HHS, OASH, OPA, *Advancing Equity in Adolescent Health through Evidence-Based Teen Pregnancy Prevention Programs and Services*, AH-TP1-23-001, 2023; (2) HHS, OAH, OPA, "Teen Pregnancy Prevention Tier 2 Adolescent Sexual Health Innovation Hubs" AH-TP2-23-002, 2023; and (3) HHS, OAH, OPA, "Teen Pregnancy Prevention Tier 2 Rigorous Evaluation Cooperative Agreements," AH-TP2-23-001, 2023.

Personal Responsibility Education Program (PREP): (1) HHS, ACF, FYSB, *State Personal Responsibility Education Program (PREP)*, HHS-2016-ACF-ACYF-PREP-1138, 2016; (2) HHS, ACF, FYSB, *FY 2024 Competitive Personal Responsibility Education Program (PREP)*, HHS-2024-ACF-ACYF-AK-0032, 2024; (3) HHS, ACF, FYSB, *Tribal Personal Responsibility Education Program for Teen Pregnancy Prevention*, Funding Opportunity Announcement and Instruction, HHS-2021-ACF-ACYF-AT-1922, 2021; and (4) HHS, ACF, FYSB, *Personal Responsibility Education Program Innovative Strategies (PREIS)*, Funding Opportunity Announcement and Instruction, HHS-2021-ACF-ACYF-AP- 1928, 2021.

Title V Sexual Risk Avoidance Education Program: (1) HHS, ACF, FYSB, *Standing Notice of Funding Opportunity for Title V State Sexual Risk Avoidance Education*, HHS-2024-ACF-ACYF-SRAE-0044, 2024; and (2) HHS, ACF, FYSB, *Title V Competitive Sexual Risk Avoidance Education (SRAE)*, HHS-2024-ACF-ACYF-SRAE-0040, 2024.

Sexual Risk Avoidance Education Program: (1) HHS, ACF, ACYF, Sexual Risk Avoidance Education Program, Funding Opportunity Announcement, HHS-2021- ACF-ACYF-SR-1927, 2021; and (2) HHS, ACF, FYSB, *General Departmental Sexual Risk Avoidance Education (GD-SRAE)*, HHS-2024-ACF-ACYF-SR-0041, 2024.

[a] The Title Sexual Risk Avoidance Education Program was known as the Title V Abstinence Education Grant program through FY2017.

[b] This law provides authority to HHS to make grants to states and other public organizations for paying part of the cost of research and demonstration projects, such as those relating to the prevention and reduction of dependency, among other related topics.

[c] See HHS, Fiscal Years 2013-2025 Justifications of Estimates for Appropriations Committee for Administration for Children and Families (PREP, Title V Sexual Risk Avoidance Education program, and Sexual Risk Avoidance Education program) and HHS, Fiscal Years 2013-2025 Justifications of Estimates for Appropriations Committee for General Departmental Management (Sexual Risk Avoidance Education program and TPP). These appropriations include sequestration for all four TPP programs in FY2013, and sequestration for PREP and Title

V SRAE (or its predecessor program, the Title V Abstinence Education Grant program) only in FY2014, FY2017, FY2022, and FY2023. The Title V Abstinence Education Grant program is the only program to have received funding prior to FY2010. In each of FY1998 through FY2009, the program received $50 million annually.

[d] The HECAT is an assessment tool to help schools and other entities identify curricula for health education courses and analyze the acceptability and appropriateness of these curricula, among other objectives. This tool addresses multiple health topics, including sexual health. Another tool cited in prior grant announcements, SMARTool, was developed by the Center for Relationship Education, a nonprofit organization, in partnership with the CDC. SMARTool is a program guide for use by schools and other entities interested in sexual risk avoidance education, and it identifies nine protective factors that help prevent sexual risk behaviors in youth.

Appendix B. Grantees Funded Under the Federal Teen Pregnancy Prevention Programs, by State

Table B-1. Federal teen pregnancy prevention programs: grantees by jurisdiction

(The table may omit grantees that are supported with program funding from prior years with project periods that include the fiscal year referenced in the column.

Some TPP grantees and PREP grantees serve youth in multiple states.)

State or Insular Area	Teen Pregnancy Prevention (TPP) Grantees in Jurisdiction (FY2023)	Type(s) of Personal Responsibility Education Program (PREP) Grants in Jurisdiction (FY2022)	Title V Sexual Risk Avoidance Education (SRAE) Grant Funding (FY2023)	GD Sexual Risk Avoidance Education Grantees in Jurisdiction (FY2023)
Alabama	No	State PREP	State Title V SRAE	No
Alaska	No	State PREP Tribal PREP	No	No

Table B-1. (Continued)

State or Insular Area	Teen Pregnancy Prevention (TPP) Grantees in Jurisdiction (FY2023)	Type(s) of Personal Responsibility Education Program (PREP) Grants in Jurisdiction (FY2022)	Title V Sexual Risk Avoidance Education (SRAE) Grant Funding (FY2023)	GD Sexual Risk Avoidance Education Grantees in Jurisdiction (FY2023)
Arizona	Tier 1 (FY2023-FY2028)	State PREP	State Title V SRAE	Yes
Arkansas	No	State PREP	State Title V SRAE	Yes
California	Tier 1 (FY2023-FY2028) Tier 2 (FY2023-FY2028)	State PREP PREIS	Competitive Title V SRAE	Yes
Colorado	No	State PREP	State Title V SRAE	Yes
Connecticut	Tier 1 (FY2023-FY2028)	State PREP	Competitive Title V SRAE	No
Delaware	No	State PREP	Competitive Title V SRAE	No
District of Columbia	Tier 2 (FY2023-FY2028)	State PREP PREIS	Competitive Title V SRAE	No
Florida	Tier 1 (FY2023-FY2028)	Competitive PREP PREIS	State Title V SRAE	Yes
Georgia	Tier 1 (FY2023-FY2028)	State PREP	State Title V SRAE	Yes
Hawaii	No	State PREP	Competitive Title V SRAE	Yes
Idaho	No	State PREP	State Title V SRAE	No

State or Insular Area	Teen Pregnancy Prevention (TPP) Grantees in Jurisdiction (FY2023)	Type(s) of Personal Responsibility Education Program (PREP) Grants in Jurisdiction (FY2022)	Title V Sexual Risk Avoidance Education (SRAE) Grant Funding (FY2023)	GD Sexual Risk Avoidance Education Grantees in Jurisdiction (FY2023)
Illinois	No	State PREP	Competitive Title V SRAE	Yes
Indiana	No	Competitive PREP PREIS	State Title V SRAE	Yes
Iowa	Tier 1 (FY2023-FY2028)	State PREP	State Title V SRAE	No
Kansas	No	Competitive PREP	Competitive Title V SRAE	No
Kentucky	Tier 1 (FY2021-FY2023)	State PREP	State Title V SRAE	Yes
Louisiana	Tier 2 (FY2023-FY2028)	State PREP PREIS	State Title V SRAE	Yes
Maine	No	State PREP	Competitive Title V SRAE	No
Maryland	Tier 1 (FY2023-FY2028) Tier 2 (FY2023-FY2028)	State PREP PREIS	State Title V SRAE	No
Massachusetts	Tier 2 (FY2023-FY2028)	State PREP	State Title V SRAE	No
Michigan	Tier 1 (FY2023-FY2028)	State PREP PREIS	State Title V SRAE	Yes
Minnesota	Tier 1 (FY2023-FY2028)	State PREP	State Title V SRAE	Yes
Mississippi	Tier 1 (FY2023-FY2028)	State PREP	State Title V SRAE	Yes
Missouri	Tier 1 (FY2023-FY2028)	State PREP	State Title V SRAE	Yes

Table B-1. (Continued)

State or Insular Area	Teen Pregnancy Prevention (TPP) Grantees in Jurisdiction (FY2023)	Type(s) of Personal Responsibility Education Program (PREP) Grants in Jurisdiction (FY2022)	Title V Sexual Risk Avoidance Education (SRAE) Grant Funding (FY2023)	GD Sexual Risk Avoidance Education Grantees in Jurisdiction (FY2023)
Montana	Tier 1 (FY2023-FY2028)	State PREP Tribal PREP	State Title V SRAE	No
Nebraska	No	State PREP	State Title V SRAE	No
Nevada	No	State PREP	State Title V SRAE	No
New Hampshire[a]	No	State PREP	Competitive Title V SRAE	No
New Jersey	Tier 2 (FY2023-FY2028)	State PREP PREIS	State Title V SRAE	Yes
New Mexico[b]	Tier 1 (FY2023-FY2028)	State PREP	State Title V SRAE	No
New York	Tier 1 (FY2023-FY2028) Tier 2 (FY2023-FY2028)	State PREP	State Title V SRAE	Yes
North Carolina	Tier 1 (FY2023-2028) Tier 2 (FY2023-FY2028	State PREP	State Title V SRAE	No
North Dakota	No	Competitive PREP	Competitive Title V SRAE	No
Ohio	No	State PREP	State Title V SRAE	Yes
Oklahoma	Tier 1 (FY2023-2028)	State PREP Tribal PREP	State Title V SRAE	Yes

State or Insular Area	Teen Pregnancy Prevention (TPP) Grantees in Jurisdiction (FY2023)	Type(s) of Personal Responsibility Education Program (PREP) Grants in Jurisdiction (FY2022)	Title V Sexual Risk Avoidance Education (SRAE) Grant Funding (FY2023)	GD Sexual Risk Avoidance Education Grantees in Jurisdiction (FY2023)
Oregon	No	State PREP Tribal PREP	State Title V SRAE	Yes
Pennsylvania	Tier 1 (FY2023-FY2028)	State PREP	State Title V SRAE	Yes
Rhode Island	Tier 1 (FY2023-FY2028)	State PREP	No	No
South Carolina	Tier 1 (FY2023-FY2028)	State PREP	State Title V SRAE	Yes
South Dakota	Tier 1 (FY2023-FY2028)	State PREP Tribal PREP	State Title V SRAE	Yes
Tennessee	No	State PREP PREIS	State Title V SRAE	Yes
Texas	Tier 1 (FY2023-FY2028) Tier 2 (FY2023-FY2028)	Competitive PREP PREIS	State Title V SRAE	Yes
Utah	Tier 1 (FY2023-FY2028)	State PREP	State Title V SRAE	No
Vermont	No	State PREP	No	Yes
Virginia	No	Competitive PREP	State Title V SRAE	No
Washington	Tier 1 (FY2023-FY2028) Tier 2 (FY2023-FY2028)	State PREP	No	No
West Virginia	Tier 1 (FY2023-2028)	State PREP	State Title V SRAE	Yes
Wisconsin	Tier 1 (FY2023-FY2028)	State PREP Tribal PREP	State Title V SRAE	No
Wyoming	No	State PREP	Competitive Title V SRAE	Yes

Table B-1. (Continued)

State or Insular Area	Teen Pregnancy Prevention (TPP) Grantees in Jurisdiction (FY2023)	Type(s) of Personal Responsibility Education Program (PREP) Grants in Jurisdiction (FY2022)	Title V Sexual Risk Avoidance Education (SRAE) Grant Funding (FY2023)	GD Sexual Risk Avoidance Education Grantees in Jurisdiction (FY2023)
American Samoa	No	No	No	Yes
Federated States of Micronesia	No	State PREP	State Title V SRAE	No
Guam	No	State PREP	Competitive Title V SRAE	Yes
Marshall Islands		No	No	No
Northern Mariana Islands	No	State PREP	No	No
Republic of Palau	No	State PREP	No	No
Puerto Rico	Tier 1 (FY2023-FY2028)	State PREP	State Title V SRAE	No
U.S. Virgin Islands	No	State PREP	Competitive Title V SRAE	No

Source: Congressional Research Service (CRS), based on U.S. Department of Health and Human Services (HHS), Office of the Assistant Secretary for Health (OASH), Office of Adolescent Health (OAH), *Current Teen Pregnancy Prevention (TPP) Program Grantees*," https://www.hhs.gov/ash/oah/grant-programs/teen-pregnancy- prevention-program-tpp/current-grantees/index.html. See also HHS, Administration for Children and Families (ACF), Family and Youth Services Bureau (FYSB), *State Personal Responsibility*

Education Program (PREP) Grantees FY2022, December 31, 2022; *Competitive Personal Responsibility Education Program (PREP) Awards FY2022*, December 30, 2022; *Personal Responsibility Education Innovative Strategies (PREIS) Program Grantees FY2022*, December 30, 2022; *Tribal Personal Responsibility Education Program (PREP) Grantees FY2022*, December 30, 2022; *Title V State Sexual Risk Avoidance Education (SRAE) Grantees FY2022,* December 30, 2022; *Title V Competitive Sexual Risk Avoidance Education (SRAE) Grantees FY2023,* February 5, 2024; and *General Departmental Sexual Risk Avoidance Education (GD SRAE) Grantees FY2023*, February 8, 2024; HHS, General Departmental Management, *Fiscal Year 2023 Justification of Estimates for Appropriations Committee*, p. 92; and HHS, Administration for Children and Families, *Fiscal Year 2023 Justification of Estimates for Appropriations Committee,* pp. 296-297.

[a] Although New Hampshire applied for State PREP funding in FY2021 and FY2022, it opted to discontinue receiving State PREP funds for FY2023. As a consequence, for FY2023, entities within New Hampshire were eligible to apply for competitive PREP funding; two such organizations were awarded competitive funds (HHS, ACF, FYSB, "Competitive Personal Responsibility Education Program (PREP) Grantees FY2023," February 5, 2024, https://www.acf.hhs.gov/fysb/grant-funding/fysb/competitive-personal-responsibility- education-program-prep-grantees).

[b] The project period for the third cohort of eight Tribal PREP grantees (in seven states) that was awarded in FY2021 is five years. However, the FY2021 Tribal PREP grant for Tewa Women United, was not continued after FY2021 (HHS, ACF, FYSB, *Tribal Personal Responsibility Education Program (PREP) Grantees FY2021,* December 30, 2022, https://www.acf.hhs.gov/fysb/grant-funding/tribal-personal-responsibility-education- program-prep-grantees).

Chapter 2

Federal Adolescent Pregnancy Prevention Programs*

Jessica Tollestrup

Background

The U.S. teen birth rate—or the number of births per 1,000 females aged 15 to 19 each year—has steadily declined since the early 1990s. The rate decreased by 78% from the most recent high of 61.8 in 1991 to the most recent low of 13.6 in 2022 (the most recent data available). Researchers suggest that multiple factors have influenced this decline; such factors may include decreasing adolescent sexual activity, particularly among younger teens, and increasing use of contraceptives among sexually active youth.

Despite the downward trend in births among youth, Congress continues to be interested in the issue of adolescent pregnancy because of associated adverse health, social, and economic challenges. Adolescent parents tend to have less education and are more likely to have low income than peers who are not adolescent parents. Children of adolescent mothers are more likely to have poorer educational and other outcomes than children of mothers who delay childbearing. Adolescent childbearing can have larger societal impacts, such as costs related to public sector health care and lost tax revenue. In addition, adolescent pregnancy rates vary substantially across racial and ethnic groups and by region. *Figure 1* displays adolescent birth rates across the 50 states; Washington, DC; and four of the insular areas in 2022. Eight states had

---

* This is an edited, reformatted and augmented version of Congressional Research Service Publication No. IF10877, updated August 22, 2024.

In: Navigating Pregnancy Challenges
Editor: Javier Giles
ISBN: 979-8-89530-857-8

the highest adolescent birth rates (20 or higher); Mississippi was the highest at 26.4. The rates for the insular areas ranged from 9.4 in the Northern Mariana Islands to 19.8 in Guam.

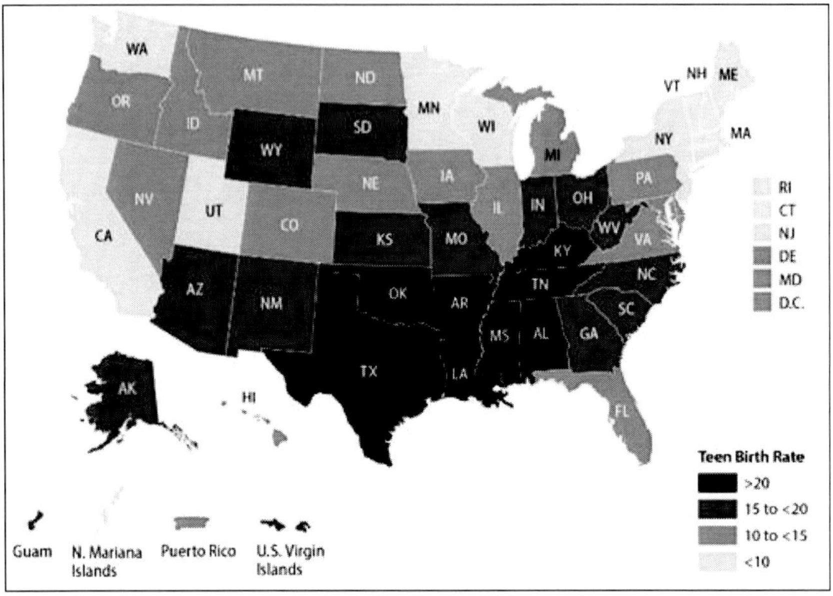

Source: Congressional Research Service (CRS), based on data from the Centers for Disease Control and Prevention (CDC).
Notes: Birth rates are per 1,000 females aged 15 to 19.

Figure 1. Teen Birth Rates by State and Territory, 2022.

Adolescent Pregnancy Prevention Programs

Federal law authorizes four federal programs that focus exclusively on adolescent pregnancy prevention education:

1) the Teen Pregnancy Prevention program;
2) the Personal Responsibility Education Program;
3) the Title V Sexual Risk Avoidance Education program, authorized under Title V of the Social Security Act (SSA); and
4) the Sexual Risk Avoidance Education program, authorized under appropriations laws. The U.S. Department of Health and Human Services (HHS) administers the four programs, which generally target

vulnerable adolescent populations. Youth receive pregnancy prevention education in schools and other settings. Grantees for the four programs include states and/or other public or private entities.

Teen Pregnancy Prevention (TPP) Program

P.L. 111-117 initially established and funded the TPP program, and subsequent appropriations laws have provided authority and funding through FY2024. The program competitively awards grants to public and private entities to implement a variety of evidence-based or innovative models that seek to influence adolescent sexual behavior. Such models focus on sexual abstinence or information about the use of contraception, among other approaches.

After funds are set aside for training and technical assistance, most of the remaining amount (75%) supports Tier 1 grants. Generally, these grantees replicate models determined to be evidence-based through rigorous evaluation studies. Another 25% of the remaining TPP program funds are used for Tier 2 research and demonstration grants. These grants are intended to develop and test additional strategies for reducing adolescent pregnancy. In FY2023, 53 Tier 1 grantees and 18 Tier 2 grants were awarded. Grantees served 140,935 youth in FY2023.

Personal Responsibility Education Program (PREP)

P.L. 111-148 established PREP under Section 513 (Title V) of the SSA. The program seeks to educate adolescents aged 10 to 20, and pregnant and parenting youth under age 21, on both abstinence and/or contraception to prevent pregnancy and sexually transmitted infections (STIs). PREP includes four types of grants: (1) State PREP grants, (2) Competitive PREP grants, (3) Tribal PREP, and (4) PREP– Innovative Strategies (PREIS). Grantees served 87,035 youth in FY2022 across all four grant types. Mandatory funding is provided through December 31, 2024.

A majority of PREP funding is allocated to states and insular areas via the State PREP grant. The 50 states, Washington, DC, and eight insular areas are eligible for funding. Funds are allocated by formula based on their relative share of youth aged 10 to 20. A total of 51 jurisdictions applied for and received FY2022 State PREP funding. Competitive PREP funding is available to local entities in jurisdictions that declined the formula grant. In FY2022, HHS noncompetitively continued grants for 27 entities to carry out PREP programming in seven jurisdictions. State PREP and Competitive PREP grantees must replicate evidence-based teen pregnancy prevention programs or substantially incorporate elements of effective programs.

Tribal PREP grants are available for tribal entities to support projects that educate American Indian and Alaska Native youth on teen pregnancy prevention. Grantees are to support culturally and linguistically appropriate teen pregnancy programs, including those that are promising or evidence-based. Seven tribal grants were noncompetitively continued in FY2022. PREIS grants are intended to build evidence for promising teen pregnancy prevention programs for high-risk youth. The grants are awarded on a competitive basis to public and private entities to implement and evaluate innovative youth pregnancy prevention strategies that have not been rigorously evaluated. PREIS supports 12 grantees in 10 jurisdictions (noncompetitively continued for FY2022).

Title V Sexual Risk Avoidance Education Program (Title V SRAE)

P.L. 104-193 established the Separate Program for Abstinence Education under Section 510 in Title V of the SSA. Now known as the Title V Sexual Risk Avoidance Education program, its purpose is to provide youth aged 10-19 with education that focuses on sexual abstinence. Any information provided about contraception is strictly limited and may not include demonstration, simulation, or distribution of contraception. Title V SRAE grantees served 240,055 youth in FY2023. As with PREP, mandatory funding for Title V SRAE is provided through December 31, 2024, with the same entities eligible to apply for Title V State SRAE funds.

States are eligible to request Title V SRAE funds if they submit an application for Title V State Maternal and Child Health (MCH) Block Grant funds. After funding is set aside for HHS administrative costs, funds are allocated to jurisdictions based on their relative shares of low-income children. A total of 38 jurisdictions applied for and received FY2023 State SRAE funding. Competitive SRAE funding is available for eligible entities in jurisdictions that do not apply for the state funds. Thirty-four Competitive SRAE grants to entities in 14 jurisdictions were awarded for FY2023. A state/territory or other entity receiving funding under the Title V SRAE program may use up to 20% of such allotment to build the evidence base for sexual risk avoidance by conducting or supporting research.

General Departmental Sexual Risk Avoidance Education Program (GD SRAE)

P.L. 114-113 established and funded the GD SRAE program, and subsequent appropriations laws have provided authority and funding through FY2024. The program supports projects for implementing sexual risk avoidance education that teaches participants how to voluntarily refrain from non-marital sexual activity and prevent other youth risk behaviors. The program targets youth populations that are at risk for non-marital sexual activity, such as juvenile justice-involved youth and youth in or aging out of foster care. HHS estimates that approximately 54,000 youth participated in the GD SRAE program in FY2019.

Multiple entities may apply for GD SRAE funding, including states and other jurisdictions such as local governments, educational, nonprofit, for-profit, and tribal entities. HHS noncompetitively continued funding for 79 grantees for FY2023. GD SRAE grantees are advised to review evidence-based program models, but do not have to use them. Prior to the GD SRAE program, appropriations laws provided funding for similar abstinence education programs, the Community-Based Abstinence Education program from FY2001 to FY2009 and the Competitive Abstinence Education program from FY2012 to FY2015. These provided competitive grants to public and private entities to develop and implement youth abstinence-only education programs.

Funding

Table 1 shows recent funding levels for the four current programs. The TPP program and GD SRAE program are supported by discretionary funds. The PREP program and Title V SRAE program are supported by mandatory funds.

Table 1. Final funding for teen pregnancy prevention programs: FY2020-FY2024 (dollars in millions)

	TPP	*PREP*	*Title V SRAE*	*GD SRAE*
FY2020	$101.0	$75.0	$75.0	$35.0
FY2021	$101.0	$75.0	$75.0	$35.0
FY2022	$101.0	$70.7	$70.7	$35.0
FY2023	$101.0	$70.7	$70.7	$35.0
FY2024	$101.0	$75.0	$75.0	$35.0

Source: CRS review of appropriations and authorizing laws.

Teen Pregnancy Prevention Evidence Review

Multiple HHS agencies established the Teen Pregnancy Prevention Evidence Review (TPPER) pursuant to P.L. 111-117. The TPPER identifies program models with statistically significant impacts on at least one of five outcomes: (1) sexual activity, (2) number of sexual partners, (3) contraceptive use, (4) STIs or HIV, and (5) pregnancies. The review was initially active from 2010 to 2019; after a pause in activity, the latest findings were released in 2023.

Some of the adolescent pregnancy prevention programs are encouraged or required to select from among the program models in the TPPER. HHS categorizes the models based on certain key features. For example, three of the models use a sexual risk avoidance approach; other models focus on healthy relationships, positive youth development, or sexual health education. The models also differ based on their outcomes, settings (e.g., schools, clinics, homes, communities), session length or duration, and target population (e.g., race/ethnicity group, age or grade level, gender, sexually active youth).

Chapter 3

Teen Birth Trends: In Brief*

Alexandria K. Mickler and Jessica Tollestrup

Summary

Adolescent childbearing is associated with significant social, health, and financial risks for teens, their families, and society more broadly. Data from the National Center for Health Statistics (NCHS), within the Centers for Disease Control and Prevention (CDC), indicate that the teen birth rate has decreased steadily over time. However, the United States continues to have one of the highest rates of teen births among other industrialized countries.

This report focuses on teen birth rates—and the marked decline in recent years. The teen birth rate is defined as the number of live births per 1,000 females aged 15 to 19 each year. The earliest NCHS estimate of the teen birth rate (in 1940) was 54.1, which later peaked in 1957 at 96.3. It then decreased in most years from the 1960s through the 1980s, with a low of 50.2 in 1986. The birth rate increased over the next few years, to 61.8 in 1991. From 1992 onward, the teen birth rate declined except in two years, 2006 and 2007. From 2007 to 2022, the rate declined by approximately 67%, to a historical low in 2022 of 13.6.

The teen birth rate has decreased across all racial and ethnic groups in recent years; however, the rates declined more for certain groups than others. From 2018 to 2022, birth rates fell by 32% for non-Hispanic Asian teens, 25% for non-Hispanic White teens, 24% for non-Hispanic American Indian or Alaska Native teens, 23% for non-Hispanic Native Hawaiian or Other Pacific Islander teens, 23% for non-Hispanic Black

* This is an edited, reformatted and augmented version of Congressional Research Service Publication No. R45184, dated August 28, 2024.

In: Navigating Pregnancy Challenges
Editor: Javier Giles
ISBN: 979-8-89530-857-8

teens, and 20% for Hispanic teens. In 2022, the teen birth rate for non-Hispanic American Indian or Alaska Native (22.5 per 1,000 females aged 15 to 19), Hispanic (21.3), non-Hispanic Black (20.3), and non-Hispanic Native Hawaiian or Other Pacific Islander (20.5) teens was more than double the rate for non- Hispanic White (9.1) teens, and more than 10 times the rate for non-Hispanic Asian (1.9) teens.

Teen birth rates have varied considerably by state and territory, which may be due to a variety of factors, such as population composition. (An analysis of these factors by state is beyond the scope of this report.) In 2022, the state with the lowest teen birth rate was New Hampshire (4.6); the state with the highest teen birth rate was Mississippi (26.4).

Thirteen states had rates of less than 10 births per 1,000 teens aged 15 to 19: New Hampshire, Massachusetts, Vermont, Connecticut, Minnesota, New Jersey, Rhode Island, Maine, New York, Utah, Washington, California, and Wisconsin (ordered from lowest to highest). Eight states had the highest teen birth rates (20 or higher): Mississippi, Arkansas, Louisiana, Kentucky, Oklahoma, Tennessee, Alabama, and Texas (ordered from highest to lowest). The rates for the territories ranged from 9.4 in the Northern Mariana Islands to 19.8 in Guam.

Teen birth rates have declined in rural areas over time but continue to remain relatively higher than teen birth rates in urban areas. The number of second (and additional) births to teen parents has also declined over time, with an 80% total decline from 2000 to 2022.

Research suggests that multiple factors have led to lower teen birth rates in the United States. From the 1990s through 2019, the risk of teen pregnancy decreased primarily because of improved contraceptive use, including an increase in the use of more effective contraceptive methods (e.g., long-acting and reversible methods) and an increase in the use of multiple methods of contraception. During this period, some of the risk of pregnancy among younger teens declined because of decreased sexual activity; however, general trends in adolescent sexual activity have remained relatively stable. Broad economic and social variables may also influence teen behaviors, such as expanded educational or labor opportunities.

Teen pregnancy has high costs for teen parents, their children, and society more generally. Teenage mothers and fathers tend to have less education and are more likely to have lower incomes than their peers who are not parents. Moreover, lower levels of education reduce teen parents' potential for economic self-sufficiency. Children of adolescent parents are also more likely to face certain adverse health and social outcomes, such as preterm birth and other child morbidities.

This report accompanies CRS Report R45183, *Adolescent Pregnancy: Federal Prevention Programs*, which discusses Congress's current approach of supporting programs that seek to prevent pregnancy among adolescents, and CRS In Focus IF10877, *Federal Adolescent Pregnancy*

Prevention Programs, which includes summary information about the programs.

Introduction

This report provides context for Congress about trends in the U.S. teen birth rate—defined as the number of live births per 1,000 females aged 15 to 19—with a focus on recent trends.[1] Since the 1950s, the U.S. teen birth rate has generally been in decline, with the rate reaching a record low in 2022 (the year for which the most recent data are available).[2] Multiple factors have likely contributed to the decrease, though the influence of any single factor is not fully understood and may vary over time. These may include proximate factors, such as contraceptive use, and distal factors, such as broader social and economic factors.[3]

Teen births are a significant public health concern because of the range of health, social, and economic effects adolescent childbearing can have on adolescents, their children, and broader society.[4] Despite substantial declines

---

[1] This report uses the terms *teenagers*, *teens*, and *adolescents* interchangeably. This report also uses *adolescent females* and *women* to be consistent with the terms used by the Department of Health and Human Services (HHS), including official teen birth statistics from the National Center for Health Statistics (NCHS). The teen birth rate age range reflects the standard definition used by the Centers for Disease Control and Prevention (CDC) and other federal agencies. The CDC also disaggregates birth rates by other age ranges, including ages 10 to 14; however, this age group is not included in calculations of the national teen birth rate and has remained unchanged since 2021 at 0.2 births per 1,000 females. See "Births: Final Data for 2022," HHS, CDC, NCHS, *National Vital Statistics Report*, vol. 73, no. 2, April 2024 https://www.cdc.gov/nchs/data/nvsr/nvsr73/nvsr73-02.pdf.

[2] In late August 2024, NCHS released a Data Brief that provides summary birth trends for 2023. The Data Brief indicates that the teen birth rate declined 4% from 2022 to 2023 to a rate of 13.1 births per 1,000 females aged 15-19. However, the Data Brief does not provide the full scope of 2023 teen birth data that are otherwise available in the "Births: Final Data for 2022" reference. As such, this report refers to final NCHS data from 2022, as it is the year for which the most comprehensive data are available. See "Births in the United States," HHS, CDC, NCHS, *NCHS Data Brief*, no. 507, August 2024 https://www.cdc.gov/nchs/data/databriefs/db507.pdf.

[3] John Bongaarts, "A Framework for Analyzing the Proximate Determinants of Fertility," *Population and Development Review*, vol. 4, no. 1 (March 1978). Laura Lindberg, John Santelli, and Sheila Desai, "Understanding the Decline in Adolescent Fertility in the United States, 2007-2012," *Journal of Adolescent Health*, vol. 59 (2016), p. 578.

[4] Urban Institute, Kids Having Kids: Costs and Social Consequences of Teen Pregnancy, edited by Saul D. Hoffman and Rebecca A. Maynard, 2nd ed., 2008. (Hereinafter, Urban Institute, Kids Having Kids: Costs and Social Consequences of Teen Pregnancy.) See also, HHS, Centers for Disease Control and Prevention (CDC), Winnable Battles Final Report 2010-2015, https://www.cdc.gov/winnablebattles/index.html; Stefanie Mollborn, "Teenage

over time, the teen birth rate in the United States has remained higher than that of comparable high-income countries.[5] Furthermore, there are persistent racial, ethnic, and geographic disparities.[6]

This report provides a description of teen birth rate trends and a brief discussion on (1) factors that may contribute to the ongoing decline in teen birth rates and (2) the adverse outcomes related to teen births. This report accompanies CRS Report R45183, *Adolescent Pregnancy: Federal Prevention Programs*, which discusses Congress's current approach of supporting programs that seek to prevent pregnancy among adolescents, and CRS In Focus IF10877, *Federal Adolescent Pregnancy Prevention Programs*, which includes summary information about the programs.

Teen Births in the United States

Official data on births to adolescent females are provided by the National Center for Health Statistics (NCHS), an agency of the Centers for Disease Control and Prevention (CDC). The NCHS, in collaboration with states and other jurisdictions, compiles and publishes official national data for all vital events (i.e., births, deaths, marriages, divorces, and fetal death) in the National Vital Statistics System (NVSS).[7] In particular, birth data in the NVSS draw upon information included in all registered birth certificates and account for nearly every birth in the United States.[8]

Data on births are distinct from data on pregnancies. Whereas the number of births—and related characteristics such as maternal age—are derived directly from vital records, information on pregnancies relies on estimates from several data sources. In addition to data on births, such figures also incorporate calculations of pregnancy losses (e.g. miscarriage, stillbirth) from the National Survey of Family Growth and estimates of induced abortion from

---

Mothers Today: What we Know and How it Matters," Child Development Perspectives, vol. 11, no. 1 (March 2017).

[5] CDC, *About Teen Pregnancy*, May 15, 2024, https://www.cdc.gov/reproductive-health/teen-pregnancy/index.html.

[6] "Births: Final Data for 2022," HHS, CDC, NCHS, *National Vital Statistics Report*, vol. 73, no. 2, April 2024 https://www.cdc.gov/nchs/data/nvsr/nvsr73/nvsr73-02.pdf.

[7] NCHS, *About the National Vital Statistics System*, https://www.cdc.gov/nchs/nvss/about_nvss.htm.

[8] NCHS estimates that more than 99% of all births occurring in the United States were registered and included in the National Vital Statistics System (NVSS). See National Center for Health Statistics, *User Guide to the 2022 Natality Public Use File*, https://ftp.cdc.gov/pub/Health_Statistics/NCHS/Dataset_Documentation/DVS/natality/ UserGuide2022.pdf.

both the CDC's Abortion Surveillance System and the Guttmacher Institute's Abortion Provider Census.[9] Various statistical approaches have been implemented over time to account for strengths and shortfalls of the aforementioned sources, as well as the inherent complexities in measuring pregnancy loss. As this report exclusively focuses on teen birth data, an evaluation of the nuances and challenges with pregnancy data are beyond the scope of this report.

Teen Birth Rate Trends

Since 1940, NCHS has published birth rate data that allow for longitudinal comparison by the age of the birth mother. The earliest estimate of the teen birth rate (in 1940) was 54.1 births per 1,000 females aged 15 to 19.[10] Twenty years later, in 1960, NCHS began publishing teen birth rate data further disaggregated by subgroups; that is, the birth rate among teens aged 15 to 17 as well as among teens aged 18 to 19. Figure 1 shows the U.S. teen birth rate from 1950 through 2022 (the rate excludes the territories).[11] Broadly, the teen birth rate (for ages 15-19) ticked up in the baby boom era of the 1950s, peaking in 1957 at 96.3. It then decreased in most years from the 1960s through the 1980s, with a low of 50.2 in 1986.[12] The birth rate increased over the next few

---

[9] Lauren M. Rossen, Brady E. Hamilton, Joyce C. Abma, et al., *Updated Methodology to Estimate Overall and Unintended Pregnancy Rates in the United States*, National Center for Health Statistics, Vital and Health Statistics: Series 2, Number 201, April 2023, pp. 1-4, https://stacks.cdc.gov/view/cdc/124395.

[10] Stephanie J. Ventura et al., "Births to Teenagers in the United States, 1940–2000," *National Vital Statistics Report*, vol. 49, no. 10, September 2001, https://www.cdc.gov/nchs/data/nvsr/nvsr49/nvsr49_10.pdf.

[11] The CDC began publishing birth rates inclusive of Alaska and Hawaii in 1959 and 1960, respectively. Data from these individuals were categorized as "Other Races," which represented a subset of the broader "Nonwhite" category historically used in earlier NVSS reports. According to the CDC, birth data from both Hawaii and Alaska affected their tabulations of birth rates by race/ethnicity in 1960, but they did not further analyze the statistical effect of this changing demographic composition among teen births, specifically. However, summary tabulations of the teen birth rate among the overarching category of Nonwhite mothers indicate a decrease in births among teens aged 10-14 and 15-19 from 1957 to 1960. This may suggest that the changing demographic composition of the United States did not significantly affect the downward trend in teen births; however, this also was not tested for statistical significance. See U.S. Department of Health, Education, and Welfare, *Vital Statistics of the United States*, Volume I - Natality, 1960, Table 1- E, https://www.cdc.gov/nchs/data/vsus/nat60_1.pdf.

[12] The baby boom era refers to individuals born in the U.S. between mid-1946 and mid-1964. Sandra L. Colby and Jennifer M. Ortman, "The Baby Boom Cohort in the United States:

years, to 61.8 in 1991. From 1992 onward, the teen birth rate declined except in two years, 2006 and 2007. From 2007 to 2022, the rate decreased by approximately 67%, with a historical low 2022 teen birth rate of 13.6.

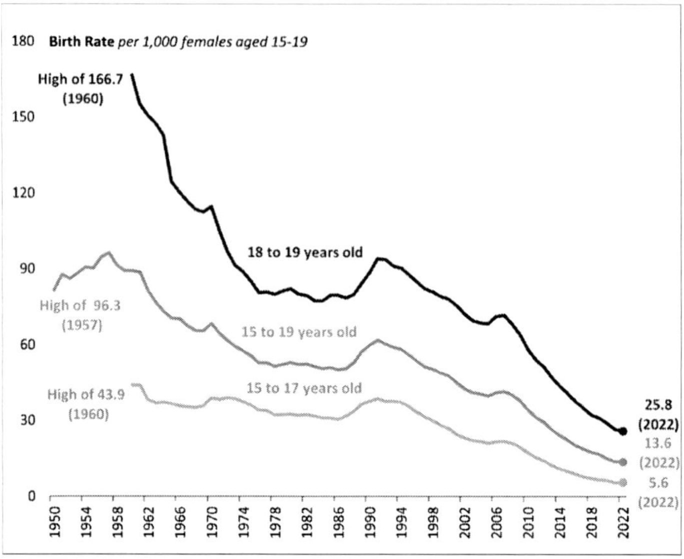

Source: Figure created by CRS using data from the following: 1950-1959 data are from Stephanie J. Ventura et al., "Births to Teenagers in the United States, 1940–2000," National Vital Statistics Report, vol. 49, no. 10, September 2001, https://www.cdc.gov/nchs/data/nvsr/nvsr49/nvsr49_10.pdf; 1960-2009 data are from Stephanie J. Ventura et al., "National and State Patterns of Teen Births in the United States, 1940–2013," National Vital Statistics Report, vol. 63, no. 4, August 2014, https://www.cdc.gov/nchs/data/nvsr/nvsr63/nvsr63_04.pdf; 2010-2020 data are from Michelle J.K. Osterman et al., "Births: Final Data for 2020," HHS, CDC, NCHS, National Vital Statistics Report, vol. 70, no. 17, February 2022, https://www.cdc.gov/nchs/data/nvsr/nvsr70/nvsr70-17.pdf; 2021- 2022 data are from "Births: Final Data for 2022," HHS, CDC, NCHS, National Vital Statistics Report, vol. 73, no. 2, April 2024 https://www.cdc.gov/nchs/data/nvsr/nvsr 73/nvsr73-02.pdf.

Notes: Subgroup data for teens aged 15-17 and 18-19 did not become available until 1960.

Figure 1. Teen Birth Rate, 1950-2022. Number of live births per 1,000 females aged 15 to 19.

2012 to 2016, Population Estimates and Projections," *Current Population Reports,* CDC, May 2014.

Recent Trends

In 2022, there were approximately 3.7 million births in the United States.[13] About 144,000 of these births (3.9%) were to teenagers aged 15 to 19. This reflects a teen birth rate of 13.6 births per 1,000 females aged 15-19 in 2022—the lowest rate on record, and a 2% decline from 2021.[14] The 2022 birth rates for 15- to 17-year-olds (5.6 per 1,000) and 18- to 19-year-olds (25.8 per 1,000) were also the lowest on record, though the birth rate among older teens remains consistently higher than the birth rate among younger teens.[15]

The 2022 rate reflects an overall decline of 67% since the most recent high in 2007 and a 78% decline from the second most recent high in 1991. In other words, about 6% of teens aged 15 to 19 gave birth in 1991 compared with less than 2% in 2022. Despite a decline in the overall teen birth rate, disparities exist among certain racial or ethnic groups. Teen birth rates in 2022 varied based on race and ethnicity, with four groups—non-Hispanic American Indian and Alaska Native (22.5 per 1,000), non-Hispanic Black (20.3), Hispanic (21.3), and non-Hispanic Native Hawaiian or Other Pacific Islander (20.5) teens—having more than double the teen birth rate for non- Hispanic White (9.1) teens, and more than 10 times the rate for non-Hispanic Asian (1.9) teens.[16]

Figure 2 shows the teen birth rate by race and Hispanic origin between 2018 and 2022. From 2018 to 2022, the teen birth rate decreased for all racial and ethnic groups; however, the rates declined more for certain groups compared with others.[17] From 2018 to 2022, birth rates fell by 32% for non-Hispanic Asian teens, 25% for non-Hispanic White teens, 24% for non-Hispanic American Indian and Alaska Native teens, 23% for non-Hispanic Native Hawaiian or Other Pacific Islander teens, 23% for non-Hispanic Black teens, and 20% for Hispanic teens. Broadly, birth rates have declined across Black, American Indian and Alaska Native, and White females; however, a

---

[13] *Table A-1* includes birth rates for teens since 1950. Michelle J.K. Osterman et al., "Births: Final Data for 2022," HHS, CDC, NCHS, *National Vital Statistics Report*, vol. 73, no. 2, April 2024, https://www.cdc.gov/nchs/data/nvsr/ nvsr73/nvsr73-02.pdf. (Hereinafter, Michelle J.K. Osterman et al., "Births: Final Data for 2022.")

[14] Ibid.

[15] The CDC also tracks births for youth aged 10 to 14. Their birth rate has been much lower than the rate of births for older teens and is therefore not included in this analysis. The birth rate was 0.2 births per 1,000 youth aged 10 to 14 in 2022, which reflects approximately 1,800 births. The 2022 birth rate for this group is unchanged from 2021.

[16] Michelle J.K. Osterman et al., "Births: Final Data for 2022," Table 2.

[17] Ibid.

1% increase in teen births was observed among Hispanic females from 2021 to 2022.[18]

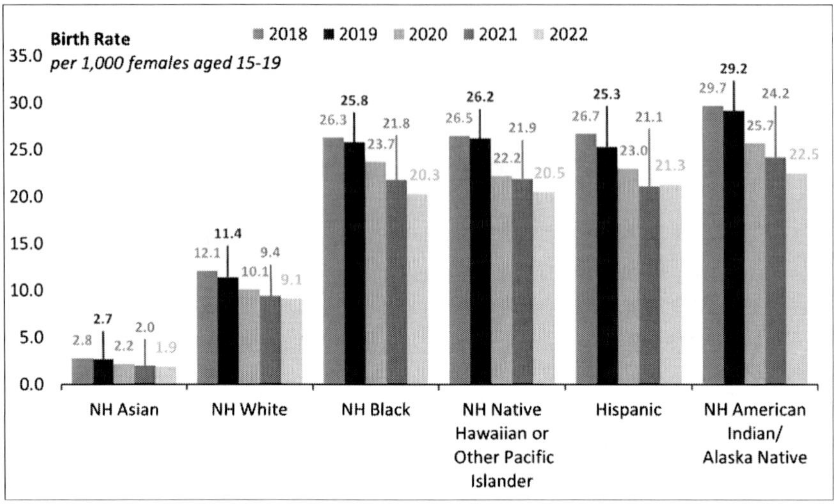

Source: Figure created by CRS using data from Michelle J.K. Osterman et al., "Births: Final Data for 2022," HHS, CDC, NCHS, National Vital Statistics Report, vol. 73, no. 2, April 2024, https://www.cdc.gov/nchs/data/nvsr/nvsr73/ nvsr73-02.pdf.
Notes: NH = Non-Hispanic.

Figure 2. Teen Birth Rate, by Race and Hispanic Origin, 2018-2022. Number of live births per 1,000 females aged 15 to 19.

Teen birth rates have varied considerably by state and territory, which may be due to a variety of factors, such as population composition. An analysis of these factors by state are beyond the scope of this report. Figure 3 shows a map of the 2022 birth rate among teens aged 15 to 19. The teen birth rate is divided into four ranges to show variations across each of the 50 states, the District of Columbia, and four of the territories.[19] The state with the lowest reported rate was New Hampshire (4.6 per 1,000); the state with the highest reported rate was Mississippi (26.4). Table B-1 in Appendix B displays the 2022 teen birth rates by state and age group.

Thirteen states had rates of less than 10 births per 1,000 teens aged 15 to 19: New Hampshire, Massachusetts, Vermont, Connecticut, Minnesota, New

---

[18] Recent changes in teen birth rates among Asian and Native Hawaiian and Other Pacific Islander females were determined to be not significant, according to the NCHS. See Michelle J.K. Osterman et al., "Births: Final Data for 2022," p. 3.

[19] Updated data were not available for American Samoa (2017 teen birth rate of 38.4).

Jersey, Rhode Island, Maine, New York, Utah, Washington, California, and Wisconsin (ordered from lowest to highest).[20] Eight states had the highest teen birth rates (20 or higher): Mississippi, Arkansas, Louisiana, Kentucky, Oklahoma, Tennessee, Alabama, and Texas (ordered from highest to lowest). The rates for the territories ranged from 9.4 in the Northern Mariana Islands to 19.8 in Guam.[21] From 2007 (when the birth rate last ticked up) to 2022, the teen birth rate decreased in each state or territory by between 58% and 78%.[22]

Teen birth rates have also declined in rural areas over time but remain relatively higher than rates in urban areas.[23]

Although the majority of teen births are first births, some teens have additional children while still in their adolescent years.[24] These births, sometimes referred to as repeat births, affect the overall teen birth rate and are associated with further risks to teen parents and their children.[25]

Recent NVSS data categorize all subsequent births as second and higher-order births (see Figure 4). Over the past approximately two decades (2000 to 2022), the rate of second and higher-order births to teens aged 15 to 19 declined by 80%, with larger declines observed among younger teenagers. The current prevalence of repeat births remains higher among non-Hispanic Black (7.0 per 1,000), Hispanic (7.1), and non-Hispanic American Indian and Alaska Native teens (8.5) compared with non-Hispanic, White teens (2.7).

---

[20] Michelle J.K. Osterman et al., "Births: Final Data for 2022," Table 8.

[21] Michelle J.K. Osterman et al., "Births: Final Data for 2022," Table 8. Data for 2022 are not reported for American Samoa (2017 teen birth rate of 38.4). Joyce A. Martin et al., "Births: Final Data for 2017," HHS, CDC, NCHS, *National Vital Statistics Report*, vol. 67, no. 8, November 7, 2018.

[22] This is based on a Congressional Research Service analysis comparing data from 2007 to 2022.

[23] Brady E. Hamilton, Lauren M. Roseen, and Amy M. Branum, "Teen Birth Rates for Urban and Rural Areas in the United States, 2007-2015," HHS, CDC, NCHS, *NCHS Data Brief*, no. 264, November 2016; and April Sutton, Daniel T. Lichter, and Sharon Sassler, "Rural–Urban Disparities in Pregnancy Intentions, Births, and Abortions Among US Adolescent and Young Women, 1995–2017," *American Journal of Public Health*, 109(12), December 2019, pp. 1762- 1769. See also Sylvester O. Orimaye, "Adolescent Birth Rates and Rural–Urban Differences by Levels of Deprivation and Health Professional Shortage Areas in the United States, 2017–2018," *American Journal of Public Health*, vol. 11, no. 1 (2021).

[24] Anne K. Driscoll et al., "Changes in First and Second Births to US Teenagers from 2000 to 2022," HHS, CDC, NCHS, *National Vital Statistics Report*, vol. 73, no. 6, July 2024, https://www.cdc.gov/nchs/data/nvsr/nvsr73/nvsr73-06.pdf.

[25] Ibid.

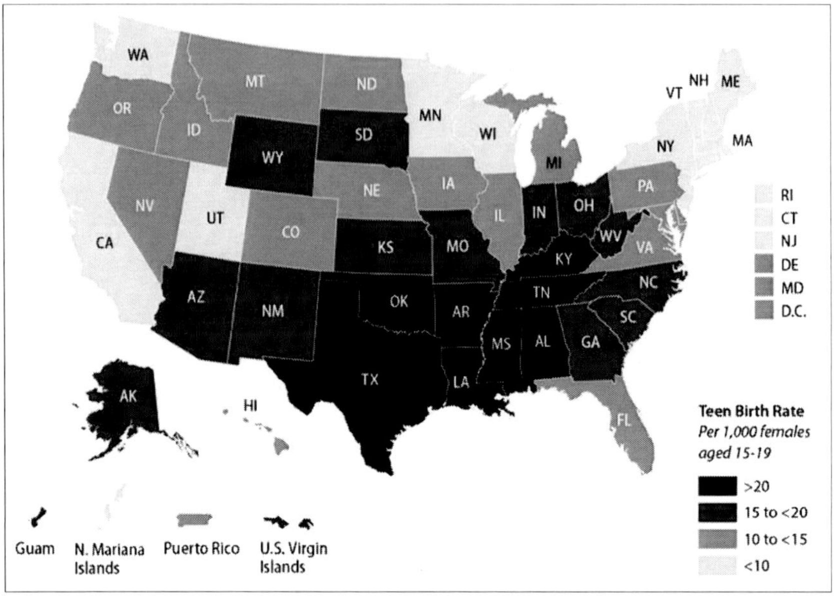

Source: Figure created by CRS using data from Michelle J.K. Osterman et al., "Births: Final Data for 2022," Table 8, HHS, CDC, NCHS, National Vital Statistics Report, vol. 73, no. 2, April 2024, https://www.cdc.gov/nchs/data/nvsr/nvsr73/nvsr73-02.pdf.

Notes: The national rate of teen births was 13.6 in 2022 (this rate does not include the territories). Data were not available for American Samoa (2017 teen birth rate of 38.4).

Figure 3. Teen Birth Rates, by State and Territory, 2022. Number of live births per 1,000 females aged 15 to 19.

Factors Linked to Declines in Teen Births

Researchers suggest that multiple factors have contributed to the near continuous decline in U.S. teen birth rates; these factors include a variety of individual, family, and broader societal factors, each of which may influence teen births to varying degrees.[26]

[26] HHS, Office of the Assistant Secretary for Health, Office of Population Affairs, "Trends in Teen Pregnancy and Childbearing," https://opa.hhs.gov/adolescent-health/reproductive-health-and-teen-pregnancy/trends-teen-pregnancy- and-childbearing.

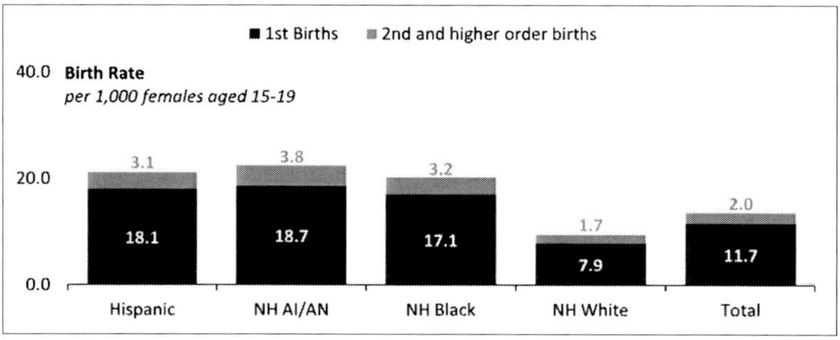

Source: Figure created by CRS using data from Anne K. Driscoll et al., "Changes in First and Second Births to US Teenagers from 2000 to 2022," Figure 2, HHS, CDC, NCHS, National Vital Statistics Report, vol. 73, no. 6, July 2024, https://www.cdc.gov/nchs/data/nvsr/nvsr73/nvsr73-06.pdf.

Notes: NH = Non-Hispanic; AI/AN = American Indian or Alaska Native. Data were not available for Asian and Native Hawaiian and Other Pacific Island groups due to (1) small numbers that prevent statistical reliability and (2) changes in how these groups were defined from 2000 to 2022.

Figure 4. First and Second and Higher-Order Teen Birth Rates, 2022. Number of live births per 1,000 females aged 15 to 19.

Over time, individual behaviors among teens have contributed to the declining teen birth rate in various manners. For instance, data from 1995 to 2002 indicated that an older age at first sexual experience accounted for 23% of the decline in teen pregnancy among younger teens (i.e., teens aged 15 to 17).[27]

More recent data indicate that trends in adolescent sexual activity have not changed significantly, but rather that decreases in the teen birth rate are attributed to an increased use of contraception.

From 2006 through 2019, teens reported an increase in the use of contraception and more consistent use of highly effective methods.[28] Teens more frequently report the use of long-acting reversible contraceptives (LARCs; e.g., intrauterine devices, or IUDs, and birth control implants), though data concerning the use of condoms remains mixed.[29] Further, the choice to

[27] Heather D. Boonstra, "What is Behind the Declines in Teen Pregnancy Rates?" *Guttmacher Policy Review*, vol. 17, issue 3, September 3, 2014, https://www.guttmacher.org/gpr/2014/09/what-behind-declines-teen-pregnancy-rates.

[28] Laura D. Lindberg, Lauren Firestein, and Cynthia Beavin, "Trends in U.S. adolescent sexual behavior and contraceptive use, 2006-2019," *Contraception X*, vol. 3 (2021).

[29] Laura D. Lindberg, Lauren Firestein, and Cynthia Beavin, "Trends in U.S. adolescent sexual behavior and contraceptive use, 2006-2019," *Contraception X*, vol. 3 (2021). See also, Leigh E. Szucs et al., "Condom and Contraceptive Use Among Sexually Active High

use certain contraceptive methods in conjunction with or instead of other methods may be influenced by a variety of factors, including clinical guidelines and related updates, physical and financial access, and individual preferences (a discussion of these influences among adolescents are beyond the scope of this report).[30] Differences in some trends in adolescent sexual behavior and contraceptive use may also depend on the sampling approach used by particular surveys.[31]

Broad economic and social variables may influence teen behaviors, such as whether they will abstain from sex or use contraceptives.[32] Behavioral changes may have been driven by a confluence of factors, such as expanded educational and labor market opportunities for women and improvements in contraceptive technology.[33] Some observers theorize that the long-term downward trend in teen birth rates is attributable to the recession that began in

---

School Students—Youth Risk Behavior Survey, United States, 2019," HHS, CDC, *Morbidity and Mortality Weekly Report Supplements*, vol. 69, no. 1 (August 2020), pp. 11-18.

[30] The CDC, as well as various independent professional membership organizations, publishes clinical guidance about the use of contraceptive methods by certain population subgroups. CDC's U.S. Medical Eligibility for Contraceptive Use (also known as the MEC) is adapted from global guidance developed by the World Health Organization. It describes who can safely use various methods of contraception based on specific health conditions and other characteristics. A companion document, known as the Selected Practice Recommendations (SPR), addresses more timely challenges regarding the initiation and/or use of certain contraceptive methods. In 2013, the SPR clarified the safety and efficacy of the use of LARC methods among adolescents, updating concerns that were previously outlined in the 2010 U.S. MEC. The 2016 update to the U.S. MEC affirmed the safety of LARC use among adolescents and women who had not previously given birth. National survey data (see footnote 29 above) indicate that adolescents used LARCs prior to these updates; however, the prevalence of LARC use has increased over time. See CDC, *U.S. Medical Eligibility Criteria for Contraceptive Use, 2016*, Morbidity and Mortality Weekly Report, July 29, 2016, pp. 4-5, https://www.cdc.gov/mmwr/volumes/65/rr/pdfs/rr6503.pdf.

[31] Laura D. Lindberg, Rachel H. Scott, Sheila Desai, et al., "Comparability of estimates and trends in adolescent sexual and contraceptive behaviors from two national surveys: National Survey of Family Growth and the Youth Risk Behavior Survey," *PLoS One*, vol. 16, no. 7 (2021). See also, Elizabeth Wildsmith, Kate Welti, Jane Finocharo, et al., *The 30-Year Decline in Teen Birth Rates Has Accelerated Since 2010*, Child Trends, December 23, 2022, https://www.childtrends.org/publications/the-30-year-decline-in-teen-birth-rates-has-accelerated-since-2010.

[32] Heather D. Boonstra, "What Is Behind the Declines in Teen Pregnancy Rates?," and Melissa S. Kearney and Phillip B. Levine, "Investigating Recent Trends in the U.S. Teen Birth Rate," *Journal of Health Economics,* vol., 41, 2015. See also, Sarah Kliff, "The Mystery of the Falling Teen Birth Rate," *Vox*, January 21, 2015. (Hereinafter, Sarah Kliff, "The Mystery of the Falling Teen Birth Rate.")

[33] Melissa S. Kearney and Phillip B. Levine, "Investigating Recent Trends in the U.S. Teen Birth Rate," *Journal of Health Economics,* vol. 41, 2015. S.M. Goodreau, "Declines in Pregnancies among U.S. Adolescents from 2007 to 2017: Behavioral Contributors to the Trend," *Journal of Pediatric and Adolescent Gynecology*, vol. 36, no. 6 (December 2022).

2007. They contend that during economic downturns the decrease in teen births—like the decrease in overall births—is partly due to teenagers being more careful as they witness the economic difficulties faced by their families.[34] Despite this rationale, the teen birth rate continued to diminish after the recession (as well as during periods of economic expansion in the 1990s).[35] Some researchers have aimed to quantify how media exposure may affect teen birth rates and related attitudes about contraceptive use and adolescent childbearing. The extent of this influence is not well understood.[36]

Some observers contend that teen pregnancy prevention programs, such as those supported with federal funding, could potentially play a role in the declining birth rate for teenagers.[37] The extent to which these programs have contributed to a decline in the teen birth rate is not fully known.[38] Some researchers have found that the proportion of teens who receive formal sex education has changed little in recent years, and that teens are less likely to be instructed on topics such as how to access contraception, how to refuse sex, and/or how to prevent sexually transmitted infections (STIs).[39] Additionally, the receipt of this information can vary by teens' sociodemographic characteristics.[40]

While the U.S. teen birth rate has decreased over time, it has been higher than that of most other industrialized countries.[41] For instance, the 2021 U.S.

---

[34] Sarah Kliff, "The Mystery of the Falling Teen Birth Rate."

[35] Melissa S. Kearney, Phillip B. Levine, and Luke Pardue, "The Puzzle of Falling U.S. Birth Rates since the Great Recession," *Journal of Economic Perspectives*, vol. 36, no. 1 (Winter 2022), pp. 151-176, and Paul Taylor, Gretchen Livingston, and Seth Motel, *In a Down Economy, Fewer Births*, Pew Research Center, Social and Demographic Trends, October 10, https://www.pewresearch.org/social-trends/2011/10/12/in-a-down-economy-fewer-births/.

[36] Melissa S. Kearney and Phillip B. Levine, *Media Influences on Social Outcomes: The Impact of MTV's 16 and Pregnant on Teen Childbearing*, National Bureau of Economic Research, Working Paper 19795, Cambridge, MA, August 2015, https://www.nber.org/papers/w19795; David A. Jaeger, Theodore M. Joycs, and Robert, "A Cautionary Tale of Evaluating Identifying Assumptions: Did Reality TV Really Cause a Decline in Teenage Childbearing?," *Journal of Business & Economic Statistics*, 38(2) (2018), pp. 317-326, https://doi.org/10.1080/ 07350015.2018.1497510.

[37] See CRS Report R45183, *Adolescent Pregnancy: Federal Prevention Programs*, for further information about current programs that are federally funded.

[38] Sarah Kliff, "The Mystery of the Falling Teen Birth Rate," and Heather D. Boonstra, "What Is Behind the Declines in Teen Pregnancy Rates?"

[39] Laura D. Lindberg and Leslie M. Kantor, "Adolescents' Receipt of Sex Education in a Nationally Representative Sample, 2011-2019," *Journal of Adolescent Health*, vol. 70 (2022), pp. 294-296.

[40] Ibid.

[41] Gilda Sedgh, "Adolescent Pregnancy, Birth, and Abortion Rates Across Countries: Levels and Recent Trends," *Journal of Adolescent Health*, vol. 56 (2015). See also Table 10 in United

teen birth rate of 13.9 per 1,000 was higher than the rate of the United Kingdom (8.2), France (5.1), Canada (4.9), and Sweden (2.5) (based on the most recent international data available that include the teen birth rate).[42] The reasons for the high teen birth rate in the United States relative to other industrialized countries have not been fully explored. Economic conditions and income inequality within and between countries, as well as societal differences, such as rates of alcohol consumption, may play a role.[43] Further, the research literature, which is somewhat limited, indicates that use of contraceptives among teens appears to be greater in other developed countries compared with the United States.[44]

Financial and Social Costs of Teen Births

Adolescent childbearing has high costs for the families of teen parents and society more generally.[45] Teenage mothers and fathers tend to have less education and are more likely to have lower income than their peers who are not teen parents. For example, approximately 90% of women who do not give

---

Nations, *Demographic Yearbook*, 71st Ed., 2020. (Hereinafter, Gilda Sedgh et al., "Adolescent Pregnancy, Birth, and Abortion Rates Across Countries: Levels and Trends.")

[42] United Nations, Statistics Division, "Demographic Yearbook 2022," https://unstats.un.org/unsd/demographic-social/ products/dyb/dyb_2022/. (See Table 10, "Live births by age of mother and sex of child, general and age-specific fertility rates: latest available year, 2013–2022.") See also, Gilda Sedgh et al., "Adolescent Pregnancy, Birth, and Abortion Rates Across Countries: Levels and Trends."

[43] John S. Santelli, Vinit Sharma, and Russell Viner, "Inequality, National Wealth, Economic Development and Global Trends in Teenage Birth Rates, 1990-2010," *Journal of Adolescent Health*, vol. 52, no. 1 (February 2013); and Melissa S. Kearney and Phillip B. Levine, "Why Is the Teen Birth Rate in the United States So High and Why Does It Matter?," *Journal of Economic Perspectives,* Spring: 26(2), 2012, pp. 141-166. (Hereinafter, Melissa S. Kearney and Phillip B. Levine, "Why Is the Teen Birth Rate in the United States So High and Why Does It Matter?"); John S. Santelli et al., "Global Trends in Adolescent Fertility, 1990–2012, in Relation to National Wealth, Income Inequalities, and Educational Expenditures," *Journal of Adolescent Health*, vol. 60, no. 2 (February 2017), pp. 161-168; and Torleif Halkjelsvik and Vegard Fykse Skirbekk, "Concurrent Decline in Teenage Fertility Rate and Binge Drinking? An Observational Study Across 45 Nations," *Drug and Alcohol Review*, 2024.

[44] Melissa S. Kearney and Phillip B. Levine, "Why Is the Teen Birth Rate in the United States So High and Why Does It Matter?" See also, Gilda Sedgh et al., "Adolescent Pregnancy, Birth, and Abortion Rates Across Countries: Levels and Trends"; Rachel H. Scott, Kaye Willings, and Laura Lindberg, "Adolescent Sexual Activity, Contraceptive Use, and Pregnancy in Britain and the U.S.: A Multidecade Comparison," *Journal of Adolescent Health*, vol. 66, no. 5 (May 2020), pp. 582-588.

[45] HHS, CDC, Winnable Battles Final Report.

birth during adolescence graduate from high school, whereas about 50% of teen mothers receive a high school diploma by 22 years of age.[46] In addition, according to the HHS Office of Population Affairs, adolescents who have children before turning 20 (compared with older parents) are

- more likely to need public assistance;
- more likely to have low income as adults; and
- more likely to have children who face challenges such as poorer educational, behavioral, and health outcomes.[47]

These adverse outcomes may be explained in part by the accompanying stressors and risk factors linked to having a child as a teen. They are also partly explained by underlying differences between those who give birth as teens and those who delay childbearing. Lower levels of education reduce teen parents' potential for economic self-sufficiency. At the same time, having lower income and less education can also increase the likelihood of teens becoming pregnant in the first place.[48] Compared with their counterparts who have children at a later age, teen mothers often come from more disadvantaged backgrounds (e.g., family more likely to receive public welfare benefits, parents have lower levels of education) or, as discussed below, may be the children of teen parents themselves.[49] In addition, teen sexual activity, even among those who do not become pregnant, can increase the risk of sexually transmitted infections (STIs), which can led to long-term health issues. Some STIs are disproportionately common among adolescents and young adults.[50]

Adolescent childbearing can also affect the children of teen parents. Children of teenage mothers have poorer outcomes than children of mothers who give birth in their early 20s or later. They are generally more likely to (1) have chronic medical conditions, (2) use public health care, (3) have lower school readiness scores, (4) do poorly in school, (5) give birth during their teen

---

[46] HHS, CDC, "About Teen Pregnancy," November 15, 2021, https://www.cdc.gov/teen pregnancy/about/index.htm.

[47] HHS, OPA, OASH, "About Teen Pregnancy and Childbearing," https://opa.hhs.gov/adolescent-health/reproductive-health-and-teen-pregnancy/about-teen-pregnancy-and-childbearing.

[48] Urban Institute, Kids Having Kids: Costs and Social Consequences of Teen Pregnancy.

[49] Melissa S. Kearney and Phillip B. Levine, "Why Is the Teen Birth Rate in the United States So High and Why Does It Matter?"; and Urban Institute, Kids Having Kids: Costs and Social Consequences of Teen Pregnancy.

[50] HHS, CDC, National Overview of STIs, 2022, January 2024.

years (females), and (6) be incarcerated (males).[51] Relatedly, NVSS data examining linked infant and maternal health records indicated that infants born to teen mothers are more likely to face higher rates of neonatal and infant mortality and morbidity, including preterm birth or low birth weight, while teen mothers also face heightened risk of maternal health complications.[52]

In addition to the consequences for teens and their families, teen childbearing has societal impacts. One study examined these societal impacts, specifically estimating the cost savings to public programs that were associated with avoiding unintended pregnancies during the teen years. The Power to Decide[53] did a simulation analysis to estimate the number of births to teenagers that had been averted due to the decrease in teen fertility rates from 1991 to 2015. The analysis then estimated total savings of $4.4 billion for this period, taking into consideration the cost savings to Medicaid that would have been associated with labor and delivery, postpartum care for the mother, and infant care, and receipt of Temporary Assistance for Needy Families (TANF), Supplemental Nutrition Assistance Program (SNAP), and Special Supplemental Nutrition Program for Women, Infants, and Children (WIC) benefits. Additional research of decreased or delayed teenage pregnancy and childbearing could help to inform the impacts for teen parents, their children, and society more generally.[54]

---

[51] Emily Holcombe, Kristen Peterson, and Jennifer Manlove, *Ten Reasons to Still Keep the Focus on Teen Childbearing*, Child Trends, March 2009; Urban Institute, *Kids Having Kids: Costs and Social Consequences of Teen Pregnancy*; and Stefanie Mollborn, "Teenage Mothers Today: What we Know and How it Matters," *Child Development Perspectives*, vol. 11, no. 1 (March 2017), pp. 63-69. See also Anna Aizer, Paul Devereux, and Kjell Salvanes, "Grandparents, Moms, or Dads? Why children of teen mothers do worse in life," *Journal of Human Resources* (November 2020), pp. 1019-1052.

[52] Ashley M. Woodall and Anne K. Driscoll, *Racial and Ethnic Differences in Mortality Rate of Infants Born to Teen Mothers: United States, 2017–2018*, National Center for Health Statistics, Data Brief, No. 371, June 2020, https://www.cdc.gov/nchs/data/databriefs/db371-h.pdf.

[53] The Power to Decide is a Washington, DC-based organization that promotes that all young people have access to the sexual health information, reproductive health services, and sense of possibility that they need—to decide if, when, and under what circumstances to get pregnant and have a child. The Power to Decide, *Progress Pays Off Savings Fact Sheet*, https://powertodecide.org/sites/default/files/media/savings-fact-sheet-national.pdf.

[54] Kelleen Kaye and Alison Ng, *Estimating the State and National Savings Associated with Declines in Teen Childbearing*, Power to Decide, January 2018. The decrease in teen births is based on the additional number of teen births estimated to have occurred in 2015 if the teen birth rate remained the same as in 1991.

Appendix A. Teen Birth Rate, 1950-2022

Table A-1. Teen birth rate, 1950-2022

Birth rate is per 1,000 females aged 15 to 19

Year	*Birth Rate*	*Year*	*Birth Rate*	*Year*	*Birth Rate*
1950	81.6	1976	52.8	2002	42.6
1951	87.6	1977	52.8	2003	41.1
1952	86.1	1978	51.5	2004	40.5
1953	88.2	1979	52.3	2005	39.7
1954	90.6	1980	53.0	2006	41.1
1955	90.3	1981	52.2	2007	41.5
1956	94.6	1982	52.4	2008	40.2
1957	96.3	1983	51.4	2009	37.9
1958	91.4	1984	50.6	2010	34.2
1959	89.1	1985	51.0	2011	31.3
1960	89.1	1986	50.2	2012	29.4
1961	88.6	1987	50.6	2013	26.5
1962	81.4	1988	53.0	2014	24.2
1963	76.7	1989	57.3	2015	22.3
1964	73.1	1990	59.9	2016	20.3
1965	70.5	1991	61.8	2017	18.8
1966	70.3	1992	60.3	2018	17.4
1967	67.5	1993	59.0	2019	16.7
1968	65.6	1994	58.2	2020	15.0
1969	65.5	1995	56.0	2021	13.9
1970	68.3	1996	53.5	2022	13.6
1971	64.5	1997	51.3		
1972	61.7	1998	50.3		
1973	59.3	1999	48.8		
1974	57.5	2000	47.7		
1975	55.6	2001	45.0		

Source: Table prepared by the Congressional Research Service based on data from the Department of Health and Human Services, Centers for Disease Control and Prevention, National Center for Health Statistics.

Notes: These data are presented in Figure 1.

Appendix B. Teen Birth Rates, by State

Table B-1. Teen birth rates, by state 2022

State/Territory	Teen Birth Rate, Total (Ages 15-19)	Teen Birth Rate, Ages 15-17	Teen Birth Rate, Ages 18-19
Alabama	20.9	9.4	37.4
Alaska	16.9	4.9	39.8
Arizona	15.1	6.0	28.8
Arkansas	24.6	9.5	48.9
California	9.8	3.8	18.9
Colorado	11.1	4.4	21.1
Connecticut	6.4	2.9	10.9
District of Columbia	12.5	7.7	16.1
Delaware	14.7	6.6	26.1
Florida	13.1	5.2	25.5
Georgia	16.6	6.6	32.5
Hawaii	11.7	3.9	24.7
Idaho	10.9	4.0	19.5
Illinois	11.3	4.4	22.2
Indiana	16.7	6.4	32.8
Iowa	12.4	5.6	22.1
Kansas	16.2	6.5	31.0
Kentucky	21.8	8.0	44.5
Louisiana	23.7	9.8	45.8
Maine	8.4	2.8	16.6
Maryland	10.9	4.8	20.4
Massachusetts	5.8	2.4	9.9
Michigan	11.6	4.4	22.6
Minnesota	8.2	3.2	16.2
Mississippi	26.4	11.6	49.1
Missouri	16.9	6.7	32.9
Montana	12.2	4.5	24.7
Nebraska	14.1	5.9	26.7
Nevada	14.0	4.8	31.0
New Hampshire	4.6	1.5	9.0
New Jersey	8.2	3.4	16.1
New Mexico	19.7	9.1	36.0
New York	8.6	3.4	15.7
North Carolina	15.0	6.5	27.1
North Dakota	11.7	4.4	20.9
Ohio	15.4	6.0	30.5

State/Territory	Teen Birth Rate, Total (Ages 15-19)	Teen Birth Rate, Ages 15-17	Teen Birth Rate, Ages 18-19
Oklahoma	21.2	8.7	40.7
Oregon	10.1	3.8	19.9
Pennsylvania	10.6	4.7	18.2
Rhode Island	8.3	3.8	13.0
South Carolina	17.3	8.3	30.3
South Dakota	17.4	7.7	32.7
Tennessee	21.0	8.4	41.6
Texas	20.4	9.0	38.6
Utah	9.0	3.1	18.1
Vermont	5.8	2.4	9.5
Virginia	11.2	4.3	31.0
Washington	9.6	3.2	20.0
West Virginia	19.8	6.7	39.3
Wisconsin	9.8	4.1	18.3
Wyoming	16.0	5.4	33.5
Total—United States	13.6	5.6	25.8
U.S. Territories			
Guam	19.8	9.0	37.1
Northern Marianas	9.4	N/A	N/A
Puerto Rico	12.6	4.4	24.7
U.S. Virgin Islands	15	N/A	29.9

Source: Figure created by CRS using data from Michelle J.K. Osterman et al., "Births: Final Data for 2022," Table 8, HHS, CDC, NCHS, National Vital Statistics Report, vol. 73, no. 2, April 2024, https://www.cdc.gov/nchs/data/nvsr/ nvsr73/nvsr73-02.pdf.

Notes: The U.S. teen birth rate does not include the territories. Data were not available for American Samoa (2017 teen birth rate of 38.4). These data are presented in Figure 3.

Chapter 4

Improving Services for Expectant and Parenting Youth in Care*

U.S. Department of Health and Human Services

Entering and navigating the child welfare system can be stressful and confusing for young people separated from their families. It can be even more challenging for young people who are parents, are pregnant, or are expecting.

Expectant and parenting youth have unique needs related to their physical, emotional, social, and financial health that require specialized support. Child welfare professionals must be well equipped to help expectant and parenting youth in care meet those needs and support them as they transition to adulthood and/or parenthood.

Lived experience leaders from FosterClub who have expertise as expecting or parenting youth in care worked in close partnership with Child Welfare Information Gateway to develop this bulletin. The experiences, insights, and advice of these young people shaped the content of this publication. When quoted, they are identified according to their preference—by name, State, or anonymous.

This bulletin provides strategies for caseworkers, agencies, and other youth-serving professionals to better support expectant and parenting youth and their families. It includes general information about working with these young people and case-level and systemwide strategies that may contribute to overall improved outcomes. This product focuses on all youth—including those who are pregnant, their partners, mothers, fathers, nonbinary parents,

* This is an edited, reformatted and augmented version of U.S. Department of Health and Human Services, Administration for Children and Families Administration on Children, Youth and Families Children's Bureau Publication, dated June 2023.

In: Navigating Pregnancy Challenges
Editor: Javier Giles
ISBN: 979-8-89530-857-8

and other members of the LGBTQIA2S+ (lesbian, gay, bisexual, transgender, questioning, intersex, asexual, Two-Spirit, or other gender or sexual identity) community.[1]

Background

All teenage and young adult parents need support, regardless of their involvement with the child welfare system. The human brain continues to develop through one's mid-20s, and adolescent and young adult brains have yet to fully develop in the areas related to reasoning, decision-making, and problem-solving. Young people expecting or parenting during this part of their lives need strong support networks and resources to become successful adults and—if they choose—parents.

Youth in foster care experience higher rates of pregnancy and parenthood compared to their peers who are not in foster care (Eastman et al., 2019). This includes both young people who become pregnant and their partners. Expectant and parenting youth in care also face unique challenges related to housing and foster care placements, completing their education, obtaining employment, understanding their parental rights, accessing health-care and mental health services, accessing child care, and more. Navigating these challenges requires specialized support from caseworkers and other professionals. However, expectant and parenting youth in care often lack the financial, emotional, social, and parenting support they need, which can lead to lower educational attainment, unemployment, homelessness, or their own children entering the child welfare system (Combs et al., 2018).

Despite the challenges and responsibilities that expectant and pregnant youth in care shoulder, they are also resilient. Being involved with the child welfare system, many of these young people are eager to give their children a childhood different from their own. Some may even benefit from the transition to parenthood as they commit to being good parents (Eastman et al., 2019). Many young parents have the resiliency and desire to succeed—they just need the help, guidance, and opportunities that every young person deserves.

---

[1] This publication aims to use inclusive language when possible, and most information applies to all expectant and parenting youth. The term "expectant" applies to youth in a partnership where one individual is pregnant. Certain sections of this publication provide information that applies to specific subsets of expectant and parenting youth, namely (1) pregnant individuals, mothers, and others who can become pregnant or give birth and (2) fathers and partners of pregnant or birthing individuals.

Working with Expectant and Parenting Youth

When working with expectant and parenting youth, caseworkers should practice meaningful youth engagement. Youth engagement occurs when caseworkers holistically partner with young people throughout their case planning and encourage them to lead discussions about their futures. It is crucial that caseworkers approach youth engagement with an attitude that values young people's active participation and inclusion. That means building relationships with youth, listening to them, and treating them as equals. To authentically engage expectant and parenting youth, caseworkers must empower youth to make their own choices and choose what goals they want to work toward as they navigate a pregnancy and/or raise a child. More information about youth engagement is available in Information Gateway's Prioritizing Youth Voice: The Importance of Authentic Youth Engagement in Case Planning.

Caseworkers should also be conscious that young parents and expectant youth in care are often faced with reconciling two conflicting identities. On the one hand, they may feel that they are still young, and on the other hand, they may experience the pressure and adult responsibilities that come with expecting and/or raising a child of their own. They often experience a similar juxtaposition in how others view them. Caseworkers, caregivers, and others may take an "adults know best" perspective and inhibit the youth from making decisions. They may also view the youth as an adult who needs to take responsibility for their actions, essentially leaving them to cope on their own.

Caseworkers need to find the right balance between treating young people as youth who need help at times and as adults with the right to make decisions. They should empower youth to take the lead in their case planning while providing the support and guidance they need to reach their goals and navigate different programs and systems. Without the right support, youth may feel overwhelmed by responsibility and feel they are left to fend for themselves. With too much input and/or oversight, youth may feel as though they are not trusted or that someone else's beliefs are being imposed upon them. Caseworkers should play a balanced role, providing support and guidance as needed while respecting a young person's wants, needs, goals, and ambitions. Caseworkers should also practice empathy and compassion, as expectant and parenting youth often experience a lot of judgment from outsiders. It is important to recognize that caseworkers cannot be the sole source of support for youth in care, so they must connect youth with peers and other supportive individuals. More information is available in this publication's Help Youth Develop Support Networks section.

The rights of expectant and parenting youth in care can be another challenge caseworkers face when working with these young people. Caseworkers should familiarize themselves with agency, county, State, and/or Tribal policies and laws related to the rights of these young people and make every effort to ensure those rights are respected. This includes their right as a parent to keep their baby in their physical and legal custody. More information about reproductive rights is available in this publication's Planning and Preparation section.

Additional guidance and resources for working with expectant and parenting youth are available on Information Gateway's Supporting Expectant, Pregnant, and Parenting Youth in Foster Care and Supporting Young Parents webpages.

> "That whole dichotomy of being a youth in care while also being a parent. . .My workers didn't know how to interact with me. At times I was punished for being a child that talked too much, and other times I was punished for being a mother that didn't do enough."—Lanitta, experienced pregnancy and parenting in foster care
>
> "Most people treat you like, 'Oh you're pregnant so you're grown now.'. . .They treat you like an adult. There is no mom figure, someone you can talk to like, 'Okay you're pregnant, let's walk you through this, blah blah blah.' It wasn't like that at all."—Jsheema, experienced pregnancy and parenting in foster care
>
> "At the end of the day I'm still a child and I need to be treated like a child in certain aspects. I still need you to hold my hand a little bit and show me, and once you see that I can ride the bike myself, you can let go."—Makaelah, experienced pregnancy and parenting in foster care

Casework Strategies for Improving Services

This section provides strategies to help caseworkers provide personalized, informed support for youth and young adults, including information about planning and preparation, accessing and connecting to resources, and developing support networks.

Planning and Preparation

Pregnancies come with many unknowns and uncertainties, especially for first-time parents and even more so for teens or young adults. When a first-time parent learns they are expecting, they might not know what a pregnancy and/or birth entails. They might not know about infant stages or child development. Young expecting parents also may feel uncertain about their future in and out of care. Establishing plans and helping young people prepare for these unknowns may help ease anxieties and set them up for success. There are various types of plans that can benefit young people: planning during pregnancy, parenting education/preparation, general case planning, and transition planning.

When a youth discloses that they are expecting, it is important that their caseworker helps them work through all their options, which usually are—and not necessarily in this order of preference—(1) proceeding with the pregnancy and raising the child, (2) proceeding with the pregnancy and arranging for the child to be adopted, or (3) terminating the pregnancy. (More information about reproductive rights, including abortion resources for those living in States where it is illegal, is available on the Planned Parenthood website.) For fathers and nonpregnant partners, caseworkers should be prepared to discuss their role in making these decisions or supporting their partner in making these decisions. Caseworkers should ensure that youth are fully informed and support them as they decide what they want to do. It is important that caseworkers and others who are substantially involved in the youth's life (relatives, foster caregivers, etc.) do not impose their personal beliefs and that they support the young person in their decision.

> "When I first became pregnant, I was very adamant to go to college and keep my baby. . .I had a plan. Unfortunately, my case manager and the other professionals on my team didn't agree with my plan. They didn't think it was possible, and they thought adoption was better. They were pushing me towards that direction, and that's what I ended up doing with my first child. And it's something that I still regret to this day."—Young person from Virginia who experienced pregnancy and parent- ing while in foster care

If they choose to proceed with the pregnancy, the young person will need prenatal care and may need help accessing affordable health care; finding an ob-gyn, midwife, or doula; and traveling to and from appointments. Other planning during a pregnancy may include the following:

- Establishing a birth plan that outlines their preferences for labor and delivery
- Signing up for pregnancy, childbirth, and/or parenting classes
- Figuring out postbirth placements

Some youth may face challenges regarding the custody of their child shortly after giving birth. Caseworkers should be knowledgeable about their State's laws—including what paperwork may be required—to prevent unnecessary separation.

When making plans during a pregnancy, it is important to ensure that both partners are actively involved in planning and decision-making, regardless of whether they are the one to give birth. The nonpregnant partner will also need support and information related to affordable health care, doctor appointments, etc. If the couple is not together, the nonpregnant partner may need legal information on their rights, including custody, child support, placement decisions, and more.

Paternity testing may also be required to establish or have a written record of the child's paternity.

Parenting education is another important form of preparation that can set expectant and parenting youth up for success. All new parents need education on how to care for a newborn and be a successful parent. Youth in care may especially benefit from parenting education because of their age and background. More information about parenting education is available in this publication's Connecting Youth with Resources section.

General case planning will look different with expectant and parenting youth since placements, permanency goals, and other factors can be impacted by the youth having a child. During case planning meetings, caseworkers should foster safe, open environments where the youth feel comfortable and have ample opportunities to ask questions and articulate their and their children's needs. The following are some questions to consider asking youth during case planning meetings to initiate important conversations:

- How will having a baby impact your placement in care? Do we need to make plans for a new placement after the baby is born?

- What role will your partner play in your child's life? Do you need to establish custody, visitation, or child support?
- How do you hope to achieve permanency? What questions do you have about reunification, guardianship, or adoption?
- What are your education and/or employment goals? What support do you need to achieve those goals?
- Do you need help obtaining child care, health care, or other support?
- How is your physical and mental health?
- How do you feel about being expectant/parenting while in care?
- Do you have a supportive adult you can talk to if you feel down or overwhelmed?
- Have you considered remaining in extended foster care after your 18th birthday (in States where it is available)?
- Have any of your goals, plans, or decisions changed since our last meeting? How can we adapt your case plan to meet your new needs?

Transition planning is vital for expectant and parenting youth who are on track to age out of the child welfare system to ensure they are prepared for independent living. Federal law requires child welfare professionals working with youth to develop transition plans at least 90 days prior to the youth turning 18. However, transition planning should be a holistic process that unfolds over several years as a young person in care approaches adulthood. For youth who are either expecting or parenting, it is especially crucial that workers put ample time and effort into preparing youth for independent living since they will be responsible for caring for and providing for a dependent. A comprehensive transition plan will address logistics such as housing, health care, education, and employment as well as psychological and emotional aspects, such as building resiliency and developing lifelong connections. In States that offer extended foster care, workers should emphasize the benefits of remaining in care after one's 18th birthday. For more information about successful transition planning, see Information Gateway's *Working with Youth to Develop a Transition Plan.*

Connecting Youth with Resources

A major element of working with expectant and parenting youth is helping them access the right resources and services. This means, first and foremost, being knowledgeable about what is available in one's State and community. It also means being able to provide referrals for organizations and programs that provide specialized support.

It is easy for youth in care to become overwhelmed by information, responsibilities, and decisions when they find out they are expecting or become a parent. If a young person does not know a resource exists, they will not be able to utilize it. It is a caseworker's job to know what resources are available, to inform the youth about them, and to help them apply for services and navigate programs. Caseworkers should work with other systems, such as health and juvenile justice systems, to take a coordinated service delivery approach when appropriate.

> "It feels like you have to have street smarts to not only know about these resources at times but be strategic with how you utilize resources and all that good stuff. I really feel like processes need to be transparent. Transparent in how you can get to those resources, transparent how to receive those resources."—Lanitta, experienced pregnancy and parenting in foster care
>
> "One thing I would say is missing from care. . .is the connection to resources. I shouldn't just hear things from word of mouth. My social worker should be equipped to be a social worker to a parenting youth. She should know what parenting classes are available to me, what cultural classes are available to me, because everyone's culture parents different."—Makaelah, experienced pregnancy and parenting in foster care

Services and resources youth may need include pregnancy resources, financial assistance, health care, mental health support, child care, parenting education, education and career resources, resources specifically for nonbirthing partners, and resources to assist with the transition to independent living.

Pregnancy resources. Young people who are expecting will likely benefit from resources designed to help them navigate a pregnancy. First-time parents especially may need information about their options, prenatal care, timelines, foods and activities to avoid, etc. Planned Parenthood and What to Expect are helpful online resource hubs for pregnancy information. When connecting youth with pregnancy resources, caseworkers should include information about less common approaches to pregnancy or childbirth, such as working with a midwife or doula or having a home birth, which may be more prevalent in other cultures.

Financial assistance. Everything from hospital and medical bills to purchasing formula and diapers to paying child support can put a financial burden on expectant and parenting youth. In addition, youth in care are often teens and young adults still in school or working low-wage jobs. Federal financial aid resources include the Special Supplemental Nutrition Program for Women, Infants, and Children (WIC), the Temporary Assistance for Needy Families program, and the Supplemental Nutrition Assistance Program, formerly known as food stamps. Other programs may also provide financial support through scholarships, subsidized child care, etc.

Health care. Caseworkers should ensure expectant and parenting youth have health-care coverage. The majority of youth in care are eligible for Medicaid (the joint Federal and State health-care program that provides coverage to low-income Americans) and can begin coverage at any time.

If a young person is already enrolled in Medicaid by the time they give birth, their newborn is automatically enrolled and remains eligible for at least a year. Information Gateway's *Health-Care Coverage for Children and Youth in Foster Care—and After* provides indepth information about eligibility pathways that enable children and youth in care to receive Medicaid, the Children's Health Insurance Program (CHIP), or other health-care coverage. More information about health care for those who are expecting or who have recently given birth is available on HealthCare.gov's Health Coverage If You're Pregnant, Plan to Get Pregnant, or Recently Gave Birth webpage.

Mental health support. An important part of health care is connecting young people with therapy and other mental health services. Expectant and parenting youth in care face the dual stressors of raising a child and being involved in the child welfare system, both of which can impact their mental health. Adolescent mothers are also more likely than adult parents to experience some degree of perinatal mood and anxiety disorder and postpartum depression (Hackett, 2020). Even with this increased need, many adolescent and young adult parents do not receive mental health services because of logistical barriers, competing priorities, stigma, negative perceptions of care, or limited availability. Left untreated, mental health disorders and challenges can leave parents without the emotional capacity to care for, talk to, comfort, and support the healthy development of their infants. Therefore, it is crucial that caseworkers are knowledgeable about the mental health services in their communities so they can connect young people with the therapy and support they need.

With access to mental health support, youth can also talk to a doctor about medications and which antidepressants and psychotropic medications are safe to take during a pregnancy. The Substance Abuse and Mental Health Services Administration has a services locator to help find providers by zip code. In addition, the National Alliance on Mental Illness has a Youth and Young Adult Resources page with guides, factsheets, videos, and more.

> "I feel like as a parenting youth, you suffer from so much trauma before you even become pregnant while in care, that's why you're in care, so I didn't really have an opportunity to have good therapy that actually taught me how to break those generational curses or cycles. I didn't have therapy that taught me not to be a toxic mom."—Makaelah, experienced pregnancy and parenting in foster care

Child care. Accessing affordable child care can be a barrier for any parent that impacts their ability to continue their education or maintain employment. Most youth in care will be eligible for subsidized child care by meeting certain income and other criteria (e.g., the primary caregiver may need to work at least 20 hours a week or be enrolled in an education program). Caseworkers should know what options are available in their State and community and help young parents apply for these programs. The Federal Office of Child Care has a locator tool with contact information for State and Territorial child care subsidy agencies.

Parenting education. All new parents need help learning how to successfully care for a newborn and raise a child. Ensuring that youth and young adults in foster care have the tools they need to be good parents may also prevent their own children from entering the child welfare system. Parenting programs for expectant and parenting youth in care may be offered by a variety of providers, including the child welfare agency, a community program, a hospital, or a school. They may come in a variety of formats, such as group classes, individual mentorships, and home-visiting programs (such as Nurse-Family Partnership, a Federal home-visiting program that connects young, first-time, low-income parents with registered nurses). Young people can often begin parenting classes during a pregnancy and continue them after their baby's birth. Effective family life education programs are typically research-backed, incorporate support from multiple sources, provide opportunities for active learning, and address the dual development of the young parent and their child (Casey Family Programs, 2018). Classes should be culturally responsive since different cultures parent differently.

Parenting education programs should also be focused on support, not surveillance.

> "There were times when if I was receiving parenting classes from the agency— or a resource from the agency that offered parenting classes— sometimes it felt directed at me in a way that criticized my parenting style instead of helping me out holistically."—Lanitta, experienced pregnancy and parenting in foster care

Education and career resources. Education and employment are key elements to setting young people on a trajectory to a successful future. However, expectant and parenting youth often face challenges (e.g., child care, finances) that make it difficult to attend classes, keep up with homework, obtain employment, and maintain a work schedule. Various education and career resources, such as scholarships, training programs, career counseling, and more, can help eliminate barriers so young people can meet their goals. Some programs, such as the New Heights Program for Expectant and Parenting Students in Washington, DC, simultaneously provide educational support and child care services so that young parents do not have to sacrifice their education to look after their children.

When helping young people pursue education or a career, it is important to recognize that everyone has different goals. These may include finishing high school, attending college, completing a GED, going to vocational school, pursuing alternative schooling, or getting a job. More information about education and employment for expectant and parenting young families is available on Youth.gov.

Resources for nonbirthing partners. Adolescent and young adult fathers and other nonbirthing partners often do not receive the same support and resources as mothers and other birth-giving parents. Further, since there are no mechanisms enforcing child welfare agencies to track and report father involvement in their children's lives, it is difficult to determine what kind of father- focused resources young fathers in foster care need (Harty & Ethier, 2022). Regardless of these gaps in research and reporting, caseworkers should treat nonbirthing partners as equals who need the same support and resources as the birth-giving parent. They will likely also benefit from resources tailored specifically to fathers and the unique challenges they face, such as navigating biases, feeling left out of parenting decisions, experiencing pressure to provide financially, etc. The National Responsible Fatherhood Clearinghouse is a good resource to share with young fathers for information about coparenting, personal resilience, child support, custody, visitation, and more.

> "There's a plethora of great information as relates to what moms need, but I think what I'm finding is that so much of what moms need, dads need, too. I find that any information that's educational around parenting, there should be something created specifically around language that supports dads. . .If dad doesn't have the things that mom has, dad can't really fully participate and engage in the rearing of his child."—Cole Williams, fatherhood practitioner and cofounder of the Delta Project, Grand Rapids, Michigan

> "I had so many outside people telling me to stop going to school, man up get a job and start working for the kid. . .It was ridiculous that people had that mindset that I need to stop school, go work and go grind. I was like, I'm not going to give up on my education because in the long run this is better for me."—Young father from Indiana who was expecting and parenting in care

Resources to help with the transition to independent living. Discussing resources should be part of transition planning so that young people can continue accessing programs and support after they leave the child welfare system. Helping youth find stable, affordable housing after they leave care is one important piece of transition planning. This includes pointing them to information they need to learn about, such as credit scores, renter's insurance, tenant rights, etc. The John H. Chafee Foster Care Program for Successful Transition to Adulthood provides assistance to help young people who are currently or formerly were in foster care achieve self-sufficiency. Activities and programs include help with education, employment, financial management, housing, emotional support, and more.

> "I personally feel like it would be helpful if before a youth ages out, the social worker or the independent living worker can have a conversation with them or show them how to utilize and obtain those resources so when they get to be 18, they're not looking like, 'Oh my god, I don't know what to do, I feel so overwhelmed.' So it really starts before they age out."—Lanitta, experienced pregnancy and parenting in foster care

See the following online resources for more information about resources for expectant and parenting youth in care:

- Resources for Expectant, Pregnant, and Parenting Youth in Foster Care (Information Gateway)
- Connecting the Dots: A Resource Guide for Meeting the Needs of Expectant and Parenting Youth, Their Children, and Their Families (Center for the Study of Social Policy)
- Resources to Help Young Parents Thrive (The Annie E. Casey Foundation)

Help Youth Develop Support Networks

All caregivers need people they can call upon when they need a supportive listener, advice, or concrete support. Unfortunately, it is common for expectant and parenting youth in care to feel isolated and alone. A lack of social support has been identified as a major issue for these young people (Eastman et al., 2019). Parenting, in general, can be isolating. The issue is exacerbated for expectant and parenting youth in care who may not have friends their age with kids or close connections with their families. In child welfare, social connection has been identified as a protective factor that makes it easier for parents to care for their children and reduces the risk of maltreatment and other negative outcomes.

Social support can come from many different avenues. It may include family, friends, partners, neighbors, teachers, coworkers, health care providers, child welfare staff, a guardian ad litem, a court-appointed special advocate (CASA), and others. When working with expectant and parenting youth in care, caseworkers should help young people identify the supportive people in their lives and facilitate regular contact so that they can develop lifelong connections that extend past their time in care.

Social networks may also include new connections with other parents formed through support groups, mentorships, or other programs. These peer-to-peer connections may be especially helpful by allowing a young person to connect with and learn from parents who are experiencing or have previously experienced a similar situation to their own. Peers who are young parents themselves can offer camaraderie, acceptance, and support. Older mentors can provide advice and coaching on parenting since many young parents in care lack adult role models. For more information, visit FosterClub's Outreach and Peer Support webpage.

> "I had a really good CASA, bless her heart, Barbara, and she was literally like my White abuelita, my White grandma, and she came in and just poured into me and watched me grow. I literally wouldn't have become a good mom at all without her. She talked to me about parenting my son and other options that I would have, putting him into school and things like that."—Makaelah, experienced pregnancy and parenting in foster care

> "I look up [parenting examples] on YouTube and TikTok—I find myself wanting to see people's daily schedules—and if I had a mentor to ask those types of questions, I think it would have put in perspective for me, what it would look like, me being in college with a baby. It would make it possible for me, because I could see someone else actually able to achieve those day-by-day goals."—Young person from Virginia who experienced pregnancy and parenting while in foster care

> "I found out about WIC and food stamps after I had my baby. When he was in the NICU [neonatal intensive care unit], the nurse who was taking care of him had told me about it and she helped me with the application and everything while I was there and before I went home. I loved my nurse."—Jsheema, experienced pregnancy and parenting while in foster care

Systemwide Strategies for Improving Services

Unfortunately, it is not uncommon for expectant and parenting youth in care to feel disappointed and let down by their experience with the child welfare system. As the system continues to evolve and improve, efforts must be made to find better ways to work with and support these young people.

Update policies and practices. A first step is updating old policies and practices and developing new ones specifically designed for expectant and parenting youth, rather than blanketing them under the same policies and practices used for the general foster care population. Because certain policies are not tailored to expectant and parenting youth, they may have unintended negative consequences.

For example, work requirements to receive certain benefits may force many young parents to choose between furthering their education and working (National Crittenton & Katcher Consulting, 2020).

Partner with those with lived expertise. A crucial element of system improvement is engaging people with lived experience and shaping policies, research, and practices based on their expertise. Children, youth, and families who have experienced the child welfare system firsthand have valuable insights into how it can improve. The voice of lived experience is important when developing policies and practices for marginalized and under-researched groups like expectant and parenting youth. Meaningful partnership goes beyond seeking input from these experts on initiatives or having them represented on committees—it involves giving children, youth, and families opportunities to be heard at all levels of policy, research, and practice and compensating them fairly for their time and expertise. More information about lived experience integration is available in the tipsheet *Building on the Lessons Learned From Division X Implementation*.

Improve data collection and utilization. Knowing about the challenges and needs of expectant and parenting youth is difficult without regularly collected, indepth data. While expectant and parenting youth in care are increasingly getting more attention as a distinct population, data about them remains limited, which makes it difficult for systems to align services with their needs and improve their and their children's overall well-being (Annie E. Casey Foundation, 2019). Even when data are collected, they may not be analyzed and leveraged for system improvement. Information to help systems leaders gather, assess, share, and leverage data on expectant and parenting youth is available in the Annie E. Casey Foundation's *Expectant and Parenting Youth in Foster Care: Systems Leaders Data Tool Kit*

Eliminate bias and stigma. Bias among child welfare professionals and service providers continues to be a systemic obstacle for expectant and parenting youth. The implicit biases of institutions and individuals based on race, ethnicity, gender identity, sexual orientation, age, geographic location, and class impact many young people and families involved with the child welfare system, including young parents and those who are expecting. On top of these institutionalized biases that exacerbate challenges, expectant and parenting youth in care face negative stereotypes and stigma associated with their group identity. For many years and in multiple contexts, these young people have been unfairly labeled by others as sexually promiscuous, irresponsible, reckless, having poor decision- making skills, lacking the capacity to parent, being absentee parents, unmotivated, bad influences, etc. (Center for the Study of Social Policy et al., 2022). They are also often subjected to narrow gender role expectations that mothers are caregivers and fathers are providers. Systems change strategies to address bias and stigma may include reframing the causes and outcomes of adolescent pregnancy and parenting, amplifying young parents' voices and positive outcomes, supporting dual transitions to adulthood and parenthood, and building young parents' protective factors.

Coordinate service delivery. The institutions that serve expectant and parenting youth in care— including child welfare agencies, community organizations, workforce development groups, and other service providers—are siloed and often fail to coordinate their services. Coordinated service delivery across systems can help parents better navigate benefits and resources without becoming overwhelmed. One option could be online and in-person resource centers that serve as "one-stop shops" for information, services, and other support.

Improve placement options. More research is needed on placement challenges for expecting and parenting youth in care. However, anecdotal evidence from young adults with experience and other subject-matter experts suggests that housing remains a major issue for these young people. This may result from placement instability, limited foster homes willing to take in a young person and their children, subpar experiences at residential home facilities, and judgment and oversurveillance from foster families and residential home staff. Systems change that could improve these challenges include increased recruitment of foster families willing to support young parents, training for families and facilities staff to reduce bias and stigma, and allocating funding for more high-quality residential home placement programs.

More information about system-level challenges that young parents experience is available in the paper *Young Parents Speak Out: Barriers, Bias, and Broken Systems* by National Crittenton and Katcher Consulting in partnership with the Annie E. Casey Foundation, which is built on interviews with young adult parents.

> "The biggest issue that pregnant and parenting youth face is agencies, partners, and other stakeholders not knowing how to interact with them in an equitable manner.
> There's a severe lack of policy that is specific to pregnant and parenting youth and what ends up happening is the default setting. . .The data that States gather for CQI (continuous quality improvement) and CFSR (Child and Family Services Reviews) processes are not adequate when it comes to reflecting pregnant and parenting youth and their needs and challenges."—Lanitta, experienced pregnancy and parenting in foster care

"Not many people want to take in someone with a child, so it's mostly group homes. And there's a lot of arguing, fights, and awkward vibes."—Young person who experienced parenting in foster care

"There was a huge stereotype of me being a single Black mother and being on government assistance. I made sure to do everything in my power to stay in my relationship with my children's father and to make sure to keep a job."—Makaelah, experienced pregnancy and parenting in foster care

Improving Two-Generation Outcomes

The children of parents with foster care experience are more likely to be placed in care than children whose parents did not experience foster care (Wall-Wieler et al., 2018; Schachter & Kroll, 2022). This is often referred to as the "intergenerational cycle of involvement with child protection services." The cycle may be perpetuated by a number of causes, including oversurveillance of young parents in care, generational poverty, lack of support, untreated mental health conditions, and other risk factors for child abuse and neglect.

It should always be the priority of the agency to keep families together. Therefore, preventing maltreatment is an important element of working with parenting youth. Under the 2018 Family First Prevention Services Act, pregnant and parenting youth are identified as a population that is eligible for Federal reimbursement for prevention services, including in-home, parent skill-based programs and mental health and substance abuse prevention and treatment services. For example, Promoting First Relationships is a nationwide home-visiting intervention and prevention program that promotes healthy relationships between children and their parents over multiple weeks and sessions. Agencies should work to specifically address expectant and parenting youth in their prevention programs, and caseworkers should be knowledgeable about prevention programs in their community.

In addition to specific prevention programs, a two-generation (2Gen) approach to supporting youth in care and their children can improve overall family well-being. While many programs and policies focus solely on the child or the parent, 2Gen approaches build family well-being by intentionally and simultaneously working with the children and the adults in their lives together since their needs are interconnected and interdependent (Ascend Aspen Institute, n.d.). These approaches often focus on improving a family's financial, social, mental, and spiritual health.

Implementing prevention strategies is important when working with expectant and parenting youth, but it is also important to recognize that sometimes intergenerational systems involvement is a result of oversurveillance, especially for families of color. Young parents in care often feel they are under constant scrutiny and need to prove their ability to parent (Wall-Wieler et al., 2018). Systemic change will require agencies and caseworkers to reevaluate the policies and practices contributing to the oversurveillance of young parents and refocus efforts on strengths-based strategies that support families before they require a child protective services investigation.

> "They weren't really trying to help me when it came to parenting. It was just like we're supposed to watch you but when it comes to how you parent, it's like we're gonna pick and prod when you're doing something wrong but we're not gonna help you to make sure you're doing something right."—Young person who experienced parenting in foster care
>
> "I honestly feel like it's really hard when you're in the system and you have a child because now you're walking on ice. It puts a magnifier on you. . .Especially as a minority, I feel like there are stereotypes and certain things that you have to do just to get by and just to make sure that you aren't upsetting the courts and it's like you're really walking on ice. To break the cycle, there needs to be some type of adjustment and bringing back not just going by the book, but looking at the situation as a human."—Young person from Virginia who experienced pregnancy and parenting in foster care
>
> "One of the reasons why families continue to be system involved is because needs continue to not be met. Allowing people the tools to be self-sufficient and giving them the space to reach permanency and stability on their terms is important. . .If this cannot happen, then the cycle will repeat."—Lanitta, experienced pregnancy and parenting in foster care

Conclusion

Youth in care experience pregnancy and parenting at higher rates than their peers who are not involved with the child welfare system, but there is a lack of policies and practices specific to these young people. These youth deserve specialized support and equitable access to resources, especially as they face bias and stigma unique to their group identity. Improving services for expectant and parenting youth requires meaningful change at the system, program, and practice level and a commitment from child welfare professionals to better support these vulnerable, resilient young people.

> "The most important thing is also creating space for healing and accountability. There are people who have a negative view of child welfare and agencies, especially people of color, growing up we were taught to hide from social workers because the department of social services was viewed as an agency that literally destroys families, so we have a negative viewpoint when it comes to agencies. What States can do is assess communities and areas that need improvement and create easier ways to rebuild relationships within the communities that they serve."—Lanitta, experienced pregnancy and parenting in foster care

References

Annie E. Casey Foundation. (2019). Expectant and parenting youth in foster care: Systems leaders data tool kit. https://www.aecf.org/resources/expectant-and-parenting-youth-in-foster-care.

Ascend Aspen Institute. (n.d.). The 2gen approach. https://ascend.aspeninsti tute.org/2gen-approach/.

Casey Family Programs. (2018). What are some strategies for supporting pregnant and parenting teens in foster care? https://www.casey.org/pregnant-parenting-teens/.

Center for the Study of Social Policy, National Council of Juvenile and Family Court Judges, & Linking Systems of Care for Child and Youth Project. (2022). Breaking the stigma and changing the narrative: Strategies for supporting expectant and parenting youth involved in systems of care. https://cssp.org/resource/breaking-the-stigma-and-changing-the-narrative-strategies-for- supporting-expectant-and-parenting-youth-involved-in-systems-of-care/.

Combs, K. M., Begun, S., Rinehart, D. J., & Taussig, H. (2018). Pregnancy and childbearing among young adults who experienced foster care. *Child Maltreatment*, 23(2), 166–174. https://doi. org/10.1177/1077559517733816.

Eastman, A. L., Palmer, L., & Ahn, E. (2019). Pregnant and parenting youth in care and their children: A literature review. *Child and Adolescent Social Work Journal,* 36(7). https://doi.org/10.1007/s10560- 019-00598-8.

Hackett, K. (2020). Addressing the mental health needs of parenting teens. PolicyLab at Children's Hospital of Philadelphia. https://policylab.chop.edu/ issue-briefs/addressing-mental-health- needs-parenting-teens.

Harty, J. S., & Ethier, K. L. (2022). Fatherhood in foster care: A scoping review spanning 30 years of research on expectant and parenting fathers in state care. *Child and*

Adolescent Social Work Journal, 39, 693–710. https://doi.org/ 10.1007/s10560-022-00848-2.

National Crittenton & Katcher Consulting. (2020). Young parents speak out: Barriers, bias, and broken systems. *PACEs Connection.* https://www. pacesconnection.com/blog/ young-parents-speak-out-barriers-bias-and-broken-systems-aecf-org.

Schachter, E., & Kroll, E. (2022). The intergenerational effects of the child welfare system and the legal obligation to rectify them. *Rutgers Journal of Law G Public Policy,* 19(2), 211–234. https:// rutgerspolicyjournal.org/2022/03/09/ intergenerational-effects-child-welfare-system-and-legal-obligation-rectify-them/.

Wall-Wieler, E., Brownell, M., Singal, D., Nickel, N., & Roos, L. (2018). The cycle of child protection services involvement: A cohort study of adolescent mothers. *Pediatrics*, 141(6). https://doi. org/10.1542/peds.2017-3119.

Suggested Citation

Child Welfare Information Gateway. (2023). Improving services for expectant and parenting youth in care. U.S. Department of Health and Human Services, Administration for Children and Families, Children's Bureau. https://www. childwelfare.gov/pubs/support-expecting-parenting/

Chapter 5

Expecting and Parenting in Care: Tips for Youth*

U.S. Department of Health and Human Services

Pregnancies and parenting come with a lot of unknowns, even for the most prepared adults. When you are expecting or parenting a child during your time in foster care, it can be challenging to balance school, work, permanency goals, and more. You deserve support as you navigate this chapter of your life, and many tools and resources are available to help.

This factsheet was developed in close partnership with lived experience leaders from FosterClub who have expertise as expectant or parenting youth in care. Their experiences, insights, and advice shaped the content in this publication. When quoted, they are identified according to their preference—by name, by State, or fully anonymous.

This factsheet has information about government assistance, parenting supports, medical services, and other resources thatmay be available to you and your family. It also has information about your options and rights when it comes to pregnancy and parenting. The information in this factsheet is for all expecting and parenting youth in care, including those who are pregnant, theirpartners, mothers, fathers, nonbinary parents, and other members of the LGBTQIA2S+ (lesbian, gay, bisexual, transgender, questioning, intersex, asexual, Two-Spirit, or other gender or sexual identity) community.[1]

---

* This is an edited, reformatted and augmented version of Factsheets for Families, U.S. Department of Health and Human Services, Administration for Children and Families Administration on Children, Youth and Families Children's Bureau, dated June, 2023.

[1] This publication aims to use inclusive language when possible, and most information is applicable to all expectant and parenting youth. The term "expectant" applies to youth in a partnership in which one individual is pregnant. Certain sections of this publication

In: Navigating Pregnancy Challenges
Editor: Javier Giles
ISBN: 979-8-89530-857-8

Pregnancy in Care

Pregnancies can be difficult to navigate, especially for first-time parents. In this section, find information about your options, health care, childbirth, and more.

Understanding Your Options

When you or your partner becomes pregnant, you face a very important decision. Usually, you will have three options to consider (not necessarily in this order of preference):

1. Parenting: Proceeding with the pregnancy and raising the child
2. Abortion: Terminating the pregnancy
3. Adoption: Proceeding with the pregnancy and arranging for the child to be adopted

If you are pregnant, deciding whether to raise a child is a very personal decision. It can be helpful to talk through your decision with your partner and others, but at the end of the day, only you can decide what is best for you. Do not let the beliefs and opinions of relatives, caseworkers, foster caregivers, attorneys, and others pressure you into making a decision that does not feel right. If you need an unbiased person to talk to about your options, you can contact your local Planned Parenthood or All-Options, a free hotline that offers peer-based counseling and support in pregnancy decision-making.

> "When I first became pregnant, I was very adamant to go to college and keep my baby. . .I had a plan. Unfortunately, my case manager and the other professionals on my team didn't agree with my plan.
> They didn't think it was possible, and they thought adoption was better. They were pushing me towards that direction, and that's what I ended up doing with my first child. And it's something that I still regret to this day."—Young person from Virginia who experienced pregnancy and parenting while in foster care

---

provide information that applies to specific subsets of expectant and parenting youth, namely (1) pregnant individuals, mothers, and others who can become pregnant or give birth and (2) fathers and partners of pregnant or birthing individuals.

If you are the partner of someone who is pregnant, it is important that you provide support during the decision-making process (and seek supports for yourself). This means being there for your partner, listening, and providing emotional and physical support.

Support can also include doing research, developing plans, and doing other thought work throughout the pregnancy. You should express your feelings and discuss your options as a team, but deciding whether to proceed with or terminate a pregnancy is ultimately up to the pregnant individual. It is important to respect and support their decision.

Since *Roe v. Wade*—the 1973 Supreme Court case that legalized abortion nationwide—was overturned in June 2022, laws about reproductive rights have become especially complicated. Many of these laws vary by State, including some requiring parental consent for abortion, which can be complicated if you are in out-of-home care. Regardless, you deserve access to safe, affordable health care, including abortion. More information about reproductive rights, including abortion resources for those living in States where it is illegal, is available on the Planned Parenthood and National Network of Abortion Funds websites. When seeking pregnancy support, be cautious of crisis pregnancy centers, which are clinics run by antiabortion activists who spread misinformation.

Paternity Testing

Paternity testing may be something either partner seeks to explore to identify or acquire an official record of paternity.

Noninvasive prenatal paternity tests can take place as early as 8 weeks after conception and involve collecting DNA samples from both people involved. These tests are usually safe and accurate. Testing can also occur after the child is born using DNA samples from the child and the alleged father.

You do not have to be the pregnant partner to request paternity testing. If you have been told you are the father of a child, but you are not sure if that's true or would like further confirmation, you can request paternity testing.

For more information, see *chapter 3* of the Office of Child Support Enforcement's *Child Support Handbook*.

Prenatal Care and Health Care

If you choose to proceed with the pregnancy, it is vital that you get prenatal care. Prenatal care ensures you and the baby stay healthy by reducing complications during pregnancy and preventing problems that can occur during delivery. It also provides opportunities to ask questions and learn about labor and delivery, breastfeeding, newborn care, and more. Prenatal appointments typically begin between week 6 and week 8 of pregnancy, start occurring monthly, and then increase in frequency as the pregnancy progresses.

When choosing an obstetrician-gynecologist (ob-gyn), some logistics to consider are the location of the practice, whether they are covered by your insurance, and the hospital where they deliver. You may also want to consider compatibility with your doctor (such as factors important to you, which could be gender, race, etc.) and your health history. (Certain conditions, such as high blood pressure, heart disease, or diabetes, may require a doctor who specializes in high-risk pregnancy.) You can find an ob-gyn near you using the search tool on the American College of Obstetricians and Gynecologists website.

You can also ask friends, family, and others you trust for recommendations. Most people chose an ob-gyn to monitor their pregnancy and deliver their baby; however, you may also choose to look for a midwife or doula.

A midwife is typically an alternative to an ob-gyn and provides support during low-risk pregnancy, labor, and delivery. They may offer a more holistic and natural approach. A doula, on the other hand, is usually used in addition to an ob-gyn or midwife and provides physical and emotional support. When looking for a midwife, doula, or ob-gyn, asking about their training, experience, and approach to pregnancy and birth may help you make a decision.

Prenatal care is typically covered by insurance, so if you don't have health-care coverage already, signing up is a good idea. Your agency and caseworker should be a source of support in ensuring you have health insurance and making sure your coverage will continue after you exit care. In addition to prenatal care, qualified health insurance plans also cover childbirth and newborn care services, which can be expensive without insurance. Most youth in foster care are eligible for Medicaid (the joint Federal and State health-care program that provides coverage to low-income Americans) and can begin coverage at any time. If you are already enrolled in Medicaid by the time you give birth, your newborn is automatically enrolled and remains eligible for at least a year. More information about health care is available in Information Gateway's Health-Care Coverage for Children and Youth in Foster Care—and After and HealthCare.gov's Health Coverage If You're Pregnant, Plan to Get Pregnant, or Recently Gave Birth webpage. If you are not sure about whether you have health-care coverage, use the following prompts to start the discussion with your caseworker:

- Do I have health-care coverage? If not, can you help me enroll?
- How does health insurance work?
- Will my health insurance cover prenatal care, childbirth, and/or newborn care? Will I be responsible for any portion of those costs?
- What financial support is available outside of insurance?

> "I would suffer without Medicaid. . . With those benefits, it really helps. It would be a hard thing right now to pay any medical bills because that's a lot of money."—Young person from Indiana who was expecting and parenting in care

If you are the partner to someone who is pregnant, it is important to stay involved during the pregnancy and maintain communication with your partner about their needs. Just because you are not carrying the baby doesn't mean you don't have a role to fill. You, too, can benefit from attending doctor appointments, understanding health insurance, learning about the pregnancy and birthing processes, and preparing for the baby's arrival. It's important that you are present and supportive for your partner. Fatherhood.gov has a list of 17 things you can do to support your partner during their pregnancy.

Labor, Childbirth, and Hospitals

Having a baby is a very personal experience, and you likely won't know exactly how labor and childbirth will unfold until it happens. Pregnancies are unique, and different hospitals and birthing centers have varying procedures, so there is no one-size-fits-all approach to childbirth. However, you and your partner can prepare for the experience by learning about labor and delivery and talking to your doctor or midwife about options ahead of time.

During pregnancy, it's a good idea to become familiar with the types of delivery (e.g., vaginal birth, c-section) and terms associated with childbirth. Prenatal appointments can be a good time to learn about the birthing process and make a plan with your pregnancy care provider for a safe delivery method. Your ob-gyn or midwife will be able to answer questions about timing, pain management, who can be in the room during the birth, special circumstances (e.g., twins), and more.

Birthing classes can also help you create a birth plan, learn about common things that may happen, and practice strategies for managing pain. Insurance may fully or partially cover the cost of these classes; you can call the customer service number on the back of your insurance card to ask what your plan covers. You may also want to ask your insurance provider about coverage related to hospital stays and bills. If paid birthing classes are not an option, there are several free childbirth videos and courses online (such as Tucson Medical Center's YouTube series, Lamaze's labor confidence course, and Pampers' nine-part childbirth series). When seeking out childbirth information online, stick to reputable sources and websites, such as hospitals and medical centers, in order to avoid misleading information.

No matter how prepared you are for childbirth, things do not always go according to plan; babies may come early or late, your ob-gyn may be on vacation, or the delivery method may need to change unexpectedly. Births can be unpredictable, but medical professionals are trained to handle these surprises and last-minute changes.

Some youth in care may face challenges related to custody and consent during or after childbirth. For example, one youth in care reported needing the consent of her foster caregiver before she could undergo an unplanned c-section, and another was told she would not be allowed to take her child home from the hospital since, as a youth in foster care, she "didn't have custody of herself." State laws related to expectant and parenting youth in care vary, and hospital staff may not be familiar with them. However, there are two important facts to remember throughout the process:

1. You have the legal right to care for your child like any other parent unless otherwise specified by a court of law.
2. Just because you are in foster care does not mean that your baby is automatically in State custody.

For more information about your rights as a parent in care, talk to your caseworker or attorney. You can also find information in the Juvenile Law

Center's resource guide on the topic. It is a good idea to talk to your caseworker or attorney about these potential custody and consent challenges as early as possible during your or your partner's pregnancy so you can be proactive and avoid potential issues.

> "The hospital got a CPS worker in my case even though there was nothing wrong. I was able to go home with my kid; they just brought me through the ringer."—Young person who experienced pregnancy and parenting in care

Additional Pregnancy Resources

- Planned Parenthood
- What to Expect

Parenting in Care

Parenting while living in out-of-home care can be a balancing act. This section contains information about government assistance, housing, education, work, parenting supports, and more.

> "Take your time. You will [mess] up and make mistakes, but you will always have tomorrow to do better. Do not allow others to dictate how you parent or love your child. You are not your parents. You got this."
> —Makaelah, experienced pregnancy and parenting in foster care

Government Assistance

There are several programs that may be available to you to help with finances and other basic needs. Your caseworker should be knowledgeable about what is available to you and help with the various application and enrollment processes. Talk to your caseworker about these and additional resources that may be available in your State and community.

- *Special Supplemental Nutrition Program for Women, Infants, and Children (WIC):* WIC is a nutrition program for infants and children up to 5 years old, as well as those who are pregnant, postpartum, and breastfeeding. To qualify, individuals must meet certain income guidelines and be determined at "nutritional risk" by a health professional. The program supplies checks, vouchers, or benefits cards to purchase specific, nutritious foods. WIC recipients can also receive nutrition education and referrals to other health services. Use this prescreening tool to see if you are eligible.
- *Temporary Assistance for Needy Families (TANF):* TANF is a program designed to help low-income families with children achieve economic self-sufficiency. Eligible recipients receive monthly cash assistance payments and other services designed to promote self-sufficiency, such as child care assistance and job preparation. Contact your State TANF program for eligibility and application information.
- *Supplemental Nutrition Assistance Program (SNAP):* Formerly known as food stamps, SNAP is the Federal nutrition assistance program that provides benefits to low-income families to purchase food. Contact your local SNAP office to apply.
- *John H. Chafee Foster Care for Successful Transition to Adulthood (the Chafee program):* The Chafee program provides youth in foster care and young adults formerly in care with services and financial assistance to help with the transition
- to adulthood. For more information, contact your State's independent living and education and training voucher coordinator.
- *Child Care Financial Assistance:* States and Territories receive Federal funding to provide child care financial assistance for low-income families. Use the Federal Office of Child Care's locator tool to get contact information for your State's child care subsidy agency.
- *Head Start and Early Head Start:* These programs help prepare children from birth to age 5 for school and provide services to help with learning, development, mental well-being, and physical health. The services are free for eligible low-income families. To find a Head Start or Early Head Start program near you, visit the Head Start program locator.

Child Support

In situations where children are living with only one parent (the custodial parent), that person can apply to receive child support payments from the child's other parent (the noncustodial parent). All States have official child support guidelines that are used to calculate how much a parent should contribute to financially support their children. To collect child support, custodial parents will need to establish a child support order. You can contact your local child support office for more information and to apply.

Housing

Some youth may be able to remain in the same out-of-home placement after their baby is born. Others may need to transfer to a kinship home, foster home, or residential care facility that is better equipped to meet the needs of a parent-baby duo. Early in your or your partner's pregnancy, talk about who the baby will live with and how it will impact your placement in care. If one of the parents does not live with the baby, they have the right to request visitation.

Your child welfare agency has an obligation to find safe and comfortable housing for you, and you deserve a say in where you and your child will live. Independent living options may be available for youth in extended foster care (youth older than 18), and some States may offer specific programs for young parents with children. Talk to your caseworker about housing during the pregnancy so you have a plan in place for when the baby comes. Your permanency goals (e.g., reunification, adoption, guardianship, transitioning to independent living) may play a role in determining the right placement for you.

If you feel as though your agency is not providing adequate support regarding housing and placement, there are steps you can take to voice your concern:

- Talk to your foster caregiver, residential home staff, or a supportive adult.
- Talk to your caseworker, their supervisor, or another member of the child welfare agency.
- Talk to your court appointed special advocate (CASA), guardian ad litem (GAL), or your State's child welfare complaint office. (More

information about the complaint process is available in the Dealing With Stigma and Oversurveillance section of this publication.)
- In case of emergency, contact 911 or the Childhelp National Child Abuse Hotline at 1-800-4-A-CHILD.

Navigating Education and the Workforce

Both pursuing education and entering the workforce are important steps young parents can take to set themselves and their families up for success. As a parent, it's important to set education and career goals that will help you financially support your family. There are different ways to provide for and support a family, and everyone has a different path. It's okay if yours does not look the same as your peers, friends, or others.

Education: Education is an investment in your future. It creates opportunities for you since many career paths require certain degrees. (It's easier to become a businessperson with a business degree or a hair stylist with a cosmetology degree.) In addition to acquiring specific career skills, education helps you develop life skills like problem solving, critical thinking, communication, and confidence. Going to school can also help you find direction in life and decide what you want to do. You can take various educational pathways, including graduating from high school, getting your GED (an alternative to the traditional high school diploma that is earned by passing an exam), going to college, or attending vocational school to learn skills in a specific trade. The Federal title IX law grants you rights and protects you from discrimination due to pregnancy or parental status in educational programs and activities. This means schools must allow you to continue participating in classes and extracurricular activities, grant excused absences and medical leave, and allow you to make up work. More information is available on the U.S. Department of Education website.

Getting a job: Entering the workforce is another path you may choose as a young parent. You may have access to workforce development programs or career counseling through your child welfare agency or community organizations and programs.

Some programs offer support with finding, applying to, and interviewing for jobs. Talk to your caseworker about your options and include "getting a job" in your case plan goals. For more information, see Information Gateway's Employment and Training Services for Youth webpage.

For young parents, balancing school or work with raising a child can be tricky. Securing reliable and affordable child care can be crucial in achieving your education and career goals. You can also tap into your support system of relatives, friends, foster caregivers, and others who may be willing to babysit and help as needed.

> "My son, he was born my finals week of senior year, and if it wasn't for how amazing my professors were and how understanding they were, it would have been really, really stressful. . .I was just thankful my professors gave us as much of an extension as a university can, that way I could graduate on time. So thankfully I did that, and what I learned from that experience is that as long as you talk and you get one person on your side, then you can get more. Don't give up, because there are a lot of people who will help you with your educational goals."
> —Young person from Indiana who was expecting and parenting in care

Even talking to your teachers or boss about your situation can be helpful. If they know you are a parent, they may be more understanding when emergencies come up. They also may be more willing to accommodate your needs, for example, by giving you an extension on an assignment because your child is sick or scheduling your work shifts around your child's daycare pick-up and drop-off times.

Young parents who need to pursue education and employment simultaneously in order to support their families may face additional challenges. These youth should also use the resources mentioned above. However, if you feel overwhelmed or struggle to juggle multiple responsibilities, talk to your caseworker about additional supports and services that may be available.

Ask your caseworker about what education and career resources may be available, such as scholarships, training programs, career counseling, and more. Some programs are specifically designed for young parents, like the New Heights Program for Expectant and Parenting Students in Washington, DC, which provides both educational support and child care services in the same location. More information about education and employment for expectant and parenting young families is available on Youth.gov.

As you think about potential careers, advocacy work may be one path you choose to pursue. As someone who experienced the child welfare system, you have valuable insights that can help the system improve. Talk to your caseworker about how you can get involved, or check out FosterClub or the

National Foster Youth Institute, two organizations that help young people get involved in child welfare reform through various programs and internships.

Being the Best Parent You Can Be

Raising children is hard, but it can be very fulfilling. It is also something that no parent can be fully prepared for. Parenting is a skill, and it takes time to find your rhythm, especially since there are multiple parenting styles and various cultures parent differently. Fortunately, there are many programs, organizations, and online resources designed to help.

> "Allowing people the tools to be self-sufficient and giving them the space to reach permanency and stability on their terms is important. On their own terms,
> meaning everybody's viewpoint of permanence looks different. My permanency values could be me going to college and finishing the business degree just like someone else's could be going to New York and going to Julliard. As long as you have an understanding and you're stable and doing what you want, and you have the ability to do so, then you have reached permanency."—Lanitta, experienced pregnancy and parenting in foster care

All new parents need help learning how to successfully care for and raise a child. Taking parenting classes can help you develop these skills. Courses usually cover things like learning about child development, communicating with your child, creating structure and rules, developing positive discipline techniques, and accessing community services. You can enroll in parenting classes through a variety of sources, including your child welfare agency, schools, hospitals, and other government and community organizations. Classes come in different formats and may be in a group setting, one-on-one, or offered via virtual learning. Home-visiting programs where nurses or other professionals help you in your home environment may also be available.

For more information and examples of parent education programs, see Information Gateway's Parent Education Programs webpage. The following are some online resources that may help:

- Young United Parents is an online resource with videos and articles on a range of parenting topics, from bathing, diapering, health, milestones, money management, self-care, and more. The website is designed to help young parents connectto and learn from a community of peers without stigma or judgement.

- National Parent Helpline is a free service that provides trained advocates to listen to you, provide emotional support, help problem solve, help connect you to services and resources, and more. The website also provides a variety of resources for parenting, basic needs, emergencies, and more.
- National Responsible Fatherhood Clearinghouse is a resource for fathers and nonbirthing parents. It provides information about strong families, healthy relationships, child support, custody, visitation, personal resilience, supporting your child in school, and more.

Another important part of being the best parent you can be is taking care of your own mental and physical health. It can be difficult taking care of another human if you are not feeling at your best physically or mentally.

Taking care of your physical health includes eating healthy, staying active, avoiding drugs and alcohol, and going to the doctor when you are sick. Taking care of your mental health and seeking out help when you need it is equally important. It's not uncommon for parents to experience depression, anxiety, and other mental health challenges. Seeking supports and services for your mental health can help improve the situation before it escalates and becomes more challenging. Talk to your caseworker about therapy and mental health services that may be available to you.

Mental health services are often covered by health insurance, and many practices offer tele-therapy and virtual options, so you don't need to worry about child care or a babysitter.

> "I never wanted to be a single mom. I never wanted that for myself, and then I became a single mom out of nowhere and I couldn't navigate. I was going through a lot of depression and anxiety. . .I know a lot of people, especially women who try to be strong, will be like, 'Oh, we got this. We can do this,' and I couldn't. I had to surrender and ask for help and reach out to friends and mentors just to say, 'I can't do this. I thought I could, but I can't.' So I got a lot of support and help."—Makaelah, experienced pregnancy and parenting in foster care

The following are some mental health resources:

- National Maternal Mental Health Hotline is a free, confidential hotline for expecting and new parents that offers access to professional counselors 24 hours a day, 7 days a week.
- FindTreatment.gov is a service locator that can help you find mental health and substance use treatment providers by zip code.
- The National Alliance on Mental Health has a Youth and Young Adult Resources page with guides, factsheets, videos, and more.

Dealing with Stigma and Oversurveillance

Unfortunately, expectant and parenting youth are often subjected to bias and stigma from adults, peers, service providers, and others.

In addition to implicit bias based on race, ethnicity, gender identity, gender expression, sexual orientation, age, geographic location, and class, you may experience negative stereotypes associated with being in foster care or being a teen or young adult parent.

One negative consequence of these unfair stereotypes is oversurveillance. You may feel as though your ability to parent is being questioned or that others are "waiting for you to mess up." Some States and agencies may even have policies and practices in place that directly subject expectant and parenting youth to increased scrutiny and supervision compared to peers who are not in the child welfare system.

One way to deal with oversurveillance is by knowing your rights. Knowledge is power, and when you are well equipped with your rights as a parent and as a youth in foster care, you can push back against unfair treatment. Two important things to know are *(1) you have the right to the legal and physical custody of your children and (2) your child is not automatically a dependent of the State just because you are.* Specific laws about your rights may vary by State, so your best bet is to talk to your caseworker or attorney about what those rights are. Some States have a foster children's bill of rights.

Another way to be proactive about oversurveillance is by keeping a detailed record of things you've done to ensure your child's safety and well-being, including a history of prenatal appointments, parenting classes, your child's doctor appointments, and more. These things can help ensure your child stays in your legal and physical custody if the State or agency petitions for removal.

If you feel as though your rights are being violated, there are steps you can take. First, talk to your caseworker, attorney, or foster caregiver. Express what feels wrong and see if you can work together to resolve the issue. If the problem is with your caseworker, contact their supervisor or someone else at the child welfare agency. Some caseworkers include their supervisor's contact information in their recorded voicemail greeting. If you have tried vocalizing your concerns and still feel unheard, contacting an ombudsman may be an option in your State. Children's ombudsman offices, sometimes known as offices of the child advocate, are offices that handle issues and complaints related to child welfare services. These offices are often separate from the child welfare agency, so you have another place to go if you feel your agency is not listening. Child Welfare Information Gateway has a list of complaint offices by State where you can see what is available where you live. For more information about resolving complaints, see Information Gateway's From Complaint to Resolution: Understanding the Child Welfare Grievance Process.

> "I would say that there are people in the system who care to help but you need to be very vocal to your workers, and if they aren't listening, ask to speak to their supervisors."
> —Young person from Indiana who was expecting and parenting in care

Planning for a Bright Future

Planning for the future may look a little different with a family since you are responsible for someone other than yourself. It's important that you are well prepared for life after the foster care system so that you have what you need to keep your family safe, happy, and healthy. If you take steps to ensure you have stable, affordable housing and continued access to resources and support, you can also help prevent your own children from entering the foster care system.

Transition Planning for Your Family

Transition planning is a process that occurs as you plan to exit out-of-home care and begin living on your own. For some youth, the transition out of foster care occurs on their 18th birthday. For others in States with extended foster care, it may occur later.

Transition planning helps you establish things like where you will live when you exit care, what education or work goals you will pursue, how you will continue accessing resources and support, and more.

Considering Extended Foster Care

In most States, you can extend your placement and continue receiving services from your social services agency after your 18th birthday. Choosing to remain in extended out-of-home care can give you more time to receive support as you prepare for the transition to self- sufficiency. Different from traditional foster care, extended care allows young people to have independence while still being able to access support. Services and resources you can receive in extended care may include academic support, career preparation, housing (traditional placements or subsidized independent living), financial assistance, mentoring, counseling, help enrolling in health care, and more. More information about extended out-of-home care is available on Information Gateway's Extending Out-of-Home Care for Youth Past Age 18 webpage.

Legally, transition planning with your caseworker must occur at least 90 days prior to your exit from care, but realistically, it should occur much sooner. As a parent, you will have a lot of decisions and logistics to navigate. The sooner you begin having these discussions about your future, the better prepared you will be, so talk to your caseworker about beginning transition planning early, even if it will be a few years before you transition out of the foster care system. When speaking with your caseworker, there are a few important topics to discuss:

- Ask about your housing options. Can you stay in your current placement? Will you need different accommodations? If you are seeking independent living, how can your caseworker help you ensure it is affordable and safe? Getting clarity on this early on will help set you up for the rest of the journey.
- Ask about resources and services available to you. Your caseworker should have some already in mind, and you can also use this factsheet as a guide to developing your own priorities. For example, what supports might you need to continue with your school and/or work

plans—child care, financial aid, transportation, etc.? If you are currently receiving services through the child welfare agency, talk about how you can apply for those services or similar ones on your own once you leave care.

Other things to consider during transition planning are independent living programs, which can help you learn about things like managing your finances, finding stable and affordable housing, developing support networks, and more. You should also make sure you leave time to collect your legal documents, such as your birth certificate, social security card, and court orders. These may be difficult to acquire once you exit State custody. For more information about the transition from care, see Information Gateway's Resources for Youth Transitioning to Adulthood webpage.

> "I personally feel like it would be helpful if before a youth ages out, the social worker or the independent living worker can have a conversation with them or show them how to utilize and obtain those resources so when they get to be 18, they're not looking like, 'Oh my god, I don't know what to do, I feel so overwhelmed.' So it really starts before they age out."
> —Lanitta, experienced pregnancy and parenting in foster care

Establishing a Support System

A significant part of preparing for the future is establishing a network of friends, relatives, and other supportive people in your life.

People need connections with other people to live happy, fulfilling lives, and we all need someone to turn to when we need help, advice, or a shoulder to cry on.

Think about the people in your life whom you trust. This may include relatives, friends, partners, neighbors, foster caregivers, teachers, coworkers, health-care providers, child welfare staff, a GAL, a CASA, and others.

Make it a priority to keep in touch with these people during and after your time in care. During your time in care, talk to your caseworker about inviting these supportive people to be part of case planning and other decision-making meetings. Having someone outside the child welfare agency with your best interests in mind can help ensure your and your family's needs are met.

Support networks don't just have to be people you already know. New connections with other parents and peers can help you find camaraderie, acceptance, and understanding from people in similar situations. These connections may be especially helpful in increasing your knowledge of how to navigate the child welfare system and better access services and supports. You may be able to make these connections through support groups and mentorships. Talk to your caseworker about what is available in your community. You can also seek out groups online or through social media.

> "Reach out for help. It doesn't make you weak; it makes you smart and stronger than those who struggle silently."—Makaelah, experienced pregnancy and parenting in foster care

Conclusion

Expecting and parenting in foster care can be difficult and isolating, but you don't have to do it alone. Use the resources in this factsheet to apply for benefits, learn about pregnancy and parenting, and set a foundation for a successful future after care. There are many programs and organizations that offer support for expectant and parenting youth, so talk to your caseworker or other adults you trust about what is available in your community.

> "I learned to not be so quick to burn bridges and build relationships with people. Learn to make mistakes while you are in care so it can be like a safety net. Explore yourself and learn how to be healed. Utilize and find all resources that are given to help you as much as you can.
> Encourage yourself to create family, friends, life goals, career paths, and overall life as you see fit."
> —Lanitta, experienced pregnancy and parenting in foster care

Additional Resources

- Resources for Expectant, Pregnant, and Parenting Youth in Foster Care (Information Gateway)
- FosterClub
- Expectant and Parenting Young Families (Youth.gov)

Suggested Citation

Child Welfare Information Gateway. (2023). Expecting and parenting in care: Tips for youth. U.S. Department of Health and Human Services, Administration for Children and Families, Children's Bureau. https://www. childwelfare.gov/pubs/expecting-parenting- youth.

Chapter 6

Education Department Updates Title IX Regulations: Protections for Pregnant Students and Employees*

Jared P. Cole
and Adam K. Edgerton

Title IX of the Education Amendments of 1972 (hereinafter, "Title IX") bars sex discrimination in education programs that receive federal financial assistance (20 U.S.C. §§ 1681 et seq.). The U.S. Department of Education's (ED's) regulations implementing Title IX cover all educational institutions that receive funding from ED programs, including all K–12 public school districts and most colleges and universities. In mid-2024, ED updated these regulations in a number of ways (34 C.F.R. Part 106). Among other things, the updated regulations define the scope of sex discrimination under Title IX to include discrimination based on sexual orientation and gender identity. They also alter the obligations for educational institutions when responding to allegations of sex discrimination, including sexual harassment. Both changes are addressed in other CRS products (see LSB11175 and LSB11200).

The updated Title IX regulations also adopt new requirements for educational institutions aimed at eliminating discrimination against pregnant students and employees. This In Focus discusses these regulatory updates.

The updated Title IX regulations took effect on August 1, 2024. However, various courts have issued preliminary injunctions against the updated regulations in their entirety. The injunctions currently cover 26 jurisdictions

* This is an edited, reformatted and augmented version of Congressional Research Service Publication No. IF12752, dated September 3, 2024.

In: Navigating Pregnancy Challenges
Editor: Javier Giles
ISBN: 979-8-89530-857-8

as well as an assortment of schools in which students or their parents are members of certain plaintiff groups. In general, the court decisions have largely focused on ED's interpretation of sex discrimination to include discrimination based on gender identity.

The Biden Administration sought to narrow the injunctions. On August 16, 2024, in a 5-4 decision, the Supreme Court denied the government's application for a partial stay of certain preliminary injunctions pending resolution of appeals in the U.S. Courts of Appeals for the Fifth and Sixth Circuits. For now, ED is barred from enforcing any portion of the updated regulations in certain states and selected schools. According to ED, the agency's prior Title IX regulations, amended in 2020, remain in place for these states and schools.

Previous Title IX Regulations on Pregnancy and Notice of Proposed Rulemaking

Prior Title IX regulations, first adopted in 1975, contained several provisions pertaining to pregnancy. For instance, they barred discrimination against students on the basis of pregnancy, childbirth, termination of pregnancy, or recovery therefrom. Educational institutions were also generally required to allow a student's leave of absence based on these conditions as long as it was deemed necessary by a physician. Further, the regulations banned discrimination in employment on these bases and required educational institutions to allow an employee's leave of absence for these conditions. (Though beyond the scope of this In Focus, employees enjoy additional pregnancy related protections under other federal statutes. For more on these laws, see CRS Report R46821, Pregnancy and Labor: An Overview of Federal Laws Protecting Pregnant Workers, by April J. Anderson.)

Following a 2022 Notice of Proposed Rulemaking, ED received comments regarding pregnancy discrimination at school. Commenters shared various experiences related to their pregnancy, including being asked to withdraw from a postsecondary institution and being excluded from school activities or programs. Commenters also noted that they had been discouraged by their educational institution from having more children, were denied accommodations generally, and often were unaware of their rights under Title IX regarding pregnancy. Some noted that when schools learn of a student's pregnancy, they may pressure the student to attend a different school of lower quality.

Another prominent concern was the lack of lactation spaces, which can impair health and interrupt learning.

Updated Title IX Regulations

In its Final Rule, ED made a number of amendments to its Title IX regulations that pertain to pregnancy. The new rule broadens the definition of pregnancy and related conditions and adds new requirements for educational institutions concerning rights for pregnant students and employees.

Scope of Protection (Definition)

The updated regulations provide that educational institutions must not discriminate based on "current, potential, or past pregnancy or related conditions." Under the regulations, pregnancy or related conditions mean pregnancy, childbirth, termination of pregnancy, lactation, related medical conditions, and recovery. The preamble to the regulations explains that the definition applies to "the full spectrum of processes and events connected with pregnancy." The preamble acknowledges that there are numerous potential medical conditions related to pregnancy, including (but not limited to) fatigue, dehydration, nausea, anemia, and prenatal or postpartum depression.

Interaction with Abortion Neutrality Provision and Religious Exemption in Title IX

While both the prior and updated regulations prohibit covered educational institutions from discriminating against students and employees based on termination of pregnancy, this requirement sits alongside two related statutory provisions in Title IX. First, the statute provides that it shall not be construed to "require or prohibit" an entity to pay or provide for a benefit or service related to abortion. The statute further provides that it shall not be construed to authorize a penalty against someone for seeking or receiving a benefit or service related to abortion. (20 U.S.C.§ 1688). In light of these provisions, the preamble to the updated regulations explains that the law does not require a campus health facility to offer abortions, nor does it require student health insurance plans to cover abortions. In contrast, educational institutions that provide health insurance for temporary conditions generally may not deny coverage for treatment of miscarriage, as that does not fall within the abortion neutrality provision's scope. The agency goes on to note that an educational institution may not retaliate against or punish a student or employee solely for seeking or obtaining an abortion. For instance, a school may not deny a student a place on the student council solely because of an abortion or deny a professor a raise on that basis.

Second, Title IX contains a religious exemption, which provides that the law shall not apply to an entity controlled by a religious organization when its application would conflict with the religious tenets of the organization (20 U.S.C. § 1681(a)(3)). The preamble to the updated regulations acknowledges that this exemption remains in place, and ED's Office for Civil Rights website appears to acknowledge exemptions from certain pregnancy requirements for religious institutions. (For more on Title IX's religious exemption, see CRS Report R47613, Title IX's Religious Exemption: Agency Practice and Judicial Application, by Jared P. Cole and Christine J. Back.)

Requirements Concerning Students

Under the updated regulations, educational institutions must ensure that when a student, or someone with a legal right to act on their behalf, informs any school employee of the student's pregnancy or related condition, the employee must promptly provide contact information for the school's Title IX Coordinator and inform the student that the coordinator can take action to ensure equal access to education programs. Once a student informs the Title IX Coordinator of their status, educational institutions must provide a general notice of nondiscrimination and inform the student of Title IX requirements regarding pregnancy, including reasonable modifications, voluntary leave, and access to a lactation space.

Educational institutions must make reasonable modifications as necessary, based on a student's individual needs, to ensure equal access to education programs.

Students have discretion to accept or decline each modification offered; if accepted, an educational institution must implement it. Reasonable modifications can include breaks during class for expressing breast milk, breastfeeding, eating, drinking, or using the restroom; intermittent absences for medical appointments; access to online classes; changes in schedules or course sequences; extensions of deadlines and rescheduling of tests; allowing a student to either sit or stand or keep water nearby; counseling; changes in space or supplies such as access to a larger desk; or other changes. Educational institutions must allow pregnant students to take a leave of absence and return to the same academic status and, as practicable, the same extracurricular status previously held.

Educational institutions must provide students with a lactation space that is not a bathroom and is clean, shielded from view, and free from intrusion. The regulations do not require that the space be any particular size or designated solely for lactation throughout the entire day.

Requirements Concerning Employees

In addition to protections for pregnant students, the updated regulations impose obligations for educational institutions with respect to employees who are pregnant.

Educational institutions must offer reasonable break time for employees to express breast milk or breastfeed. They must ensure that employees also have access to a lactation space that is not a bathroom and is clean, shielded from view, and free from intrusion. However, unlike relevant obligations for pregnant students, the Title IX regulations do not require reasonable workplace modifications that are based on an employee's individual needs (although, as mentioned above, other federal laws may do so).

Selected Bills in Recent Congresses

Two bills since 2019 have sought to address the rights of pregnant students outside of the Title IX rulemaking context. H.R. 6914 in the 118th Congress, which has passed the House, would require all institutions of higher education (IHEs) participating in the federal student aid programs authorized under Title IV of the Higher Education Act (HEA) to provide information on resources available to help pregnant students "carry the baby to term and parent the baby after birth." In the 116th Congress, H.R. 5222 would have required each IHE participating in the HEA Title IV federal student aid programs to publish expectant parent and parenting student policies, which would have included information on accommodations.

At least one congressional measure aims to oppose the updated regulations. The Congressional Review Act (CRA) establishes procedures to enact a joint resolution of disapproval that will render a regulation ineffective if passed by both houses and signed by the President (or if Congress overrides a veto). Pursuant to the CRA, H.J.Res. 165, which passed the House on July 11, 2024, would overturn the Final Rule and prohibit the Administration from reissuing the rule "in a substantially similar form" or from issuing a "new rule that is substantially the same" unless "the reissued or new rule is specifically authorized" by a later enacted law.

Chapter 7

Pregnant Students' Rights Act*

Committee on Education and the Workforce

The Committee on Education and the Workforce, to whom was referred the bill (H.R. 6914) to require institutions of higher education to disseminate information on the rights of, and accommodations and resources for, pregnant students, and for other purposes, having considered the same, reports favorably thereon with an amendment and recommends that the bill as amended do pass.

The amendment is as follows:

Strike all after the enacting clause and insert the following:

SECTION 1. SHORT TITLE.

This Act may be cited as the "Pregnant Students' Rights Act."

SEC. 2. FINDINGS.

Congress finds the following:

(1) Female students enrolled at institutions of higher education and experiencing an unplanned pregnancy may face pressure that their only option is to receive an abortion or risk academic failure.

(2) Almost 30 percent of all abortions in the United States are performed on women of college age, between the ages of 20 and 24, according to a 2021 report by the Centers for Disease Control and Prevention.

(3) Scientific evidence and personal testimonies document that women who have abortions can be at risk of mental health issues. Studies show that after an abortion, women are 34 percent more likely to develop anxiety disorders, 37 percent more likely to develop depression, 110 percent more

* This is an edited, reformatted and augmented version of Report of Ms. FOXX from the Committee on Education and the Workforce, committed to the Committee of the Whole House on the State of the Union and ordered to be printed, Publication No. 118–344, dated January 12, 2024.

In: Navigating Pregnancy Challenges
Editor: Javier Giles
ISBN: 979-8-89530-857-8

likely to rely on alcohol use or abuse, 115 percent more likely to develop suicidal behavior, and 220 percent more likely to take on marijuana use or abuse. As many as 60 percent of women having an abortion experience some level of emotional distress 49–006. afterwards, with 30 percent being classified as severe distress. Potential complications of abortions include heavy or persistent bleeding, damage to cervix, abdominal pain or cramping, scarring of uterine lining, breast cancer, future premature births or miscarriages, infection or sepsis, placenta previa, perforation of uterus, damage to other organs, and even death.

(4) A significant proportion of abortions in the United States are performed on women of college age who may be unaware of their rights to accommodation and prohibitions against discrimination due to pregnancy under title IX of the Education Amendments of 1972 (20 U.S.C. 1681 et seq.) or deprived of information about abortion alternatives.

(5) Additionally, women on college campuses may fear institutional reprisal, loss of athletic scholarship, and possible negative impact on academic opportunities during the pregnancy and after childbirth.

(6) An academic disparity exists because of the lack of resources, support, and notifications available for female college students who do not wish to receive an abortion or who carry their unborn babies to term.

SEC. 3. NOTICE OF PREGNANT STUDENT RIGHTS, ACCOMMODATIONS, AND RESOURCES.

Section 485 of the Higher Education Act of 1965 (20 U.S.C. 1092) is amended by adding at the end the following:

"(n) PREGNANT STUDENTS' RIGHTS, ACCOMMODATIONS, AND RESOURCES. —

"(1) IN GENERAL.— Each institution of higher education participating in any program under this title shall carry out the information dissemination activities described in paragraph (3) for prospective and enrolled students (including those attending or planning to attend less than full time) regarding the information described in paragraph (2) on the rights to, and resources (including protections and accommodations) for, pregnant students to carry a baby to term and students who may become pregnant while enrolled at such institution of higher education to carry a baby to term.

"(2) INFORMATION CONTENT. — The information described in this paragraph is the following:

"(A) A list of resources on campus and in the community that exist to help a pregnant student in carrying the baby to term and caring for the baby after birth.

"(B) Information about the accommodations available to help a pregnant student carry the baby to term and parent the baby after birth.

"(C) Information on how to file a complaint with—

"(i) the Department of Education, if a student believes there was a violation by the institution of title IX of the Education Amendments of 1972 (20 U.S.C. 1681 et seq.) on account of such student's determination to carry a baby to term; and

"(ii) the institution, if a student believes the student has been discriminated against in violation of such title IX on account of the student's determination to carry a baby to term.

"(3) INFORMATION DISSEMINATION ACTIVITIES. — The information dissemination activities described in this paragraph shall include—

"(A) an email to each enrolled student at the start of each period of study during an academic year; and

"(B) the provision of information— "(i) in student handbooks, if any;

"(ii) at each orientation for enrolled students;

"(iii) at student health or counseling centers, if any; and

"(iv) on the publicly available website of the institution of higher education.

"(4) RULE OF CONSTRUCTION. — Nothing in this subsection shall be construed to authorize the Secretary to require the dissemination of additional information, or establish additional rights, beyond the information and rights included in this subsection."

Purpose

The purpose of H.R. 6914, the Pregnant Students' Rights Act, is to require institutions of higher education to disseminate information on the rights of, and accommodations and resources for, pregnant students to carry a baby to term.

Committee Action

118TH CONGRESS
First Session—Hearings

On May 16, 2023, the Committee on Education and the Workforce held a hearing on "Examining the Policies and Priorities of the U.S. Department of Education." The purpose of the hearing was to examine the policies and the budget priorities of the U.S. Department of Education. During the hearing, Representative Aaron Bean (R–FL), when questioning Secretary Cardona, stated that policies need to be created to help non-traditional students, specifically single mothers, complete their postsecondary education. Testifying before the Committee was Miguel Cardona, Secretary, U.S. Department of Education, Washington, DC.

On June 14, 2023, the Subcommittee on Higher Education and Workforce Development held a hearing on "Postsecondary Innovation: Preparing Today's Students for Tomorrow's Opportunities." During the hearing, Subcommittee Chairman Burgess Owens (R– UT) identified lingering issues that non-traditional students face. Testifying before the Committee were Dr. Tim Renick, Executive Director, National Institute for Student Success, Georgia State University, Atlanta, GA; Mr. Keith Shoates, Chief Operating Officer, Student Freedom Initiative, Washington, DC; Ms. Lanae Erickson, Senior Vice President for Social Policy, Education and Politics, Third Way, Washington, DC; Dr. Lori Carrell, Chancellor, University of Minnesota Rochester and Co-Director, College-in-3 Initiative, Rochester, MN.

Legislative Action

On January 5, 2024, Representative Ashley Hinson (R–IA) introduced H.R. 6914, the Pregnant Students' Rights Act. The bill was referred solely to the Committee on Education and the Workforce. On January 10, 2024, the Committee considered H.R. 6914 in legislative session and reported it favorably, as amended, to the House of Representatives by a recorded vote of 24 yeas and 17 nays. The Committee considered the following amendments to H.R. 6914:

1. Amendment in the Nature of a Substitute—Representative Mary Miller (R–IL) offered an Amendment in the Nature of a Substitute (ANS) that further clarifies that the purpose of the required information dissemination is to support pregnant students carrying a pregnancy to term. The substitute amendment also adds a rule of construction to prohibit the Secretary from requiring institutions to disseminate additional information or establish additional rights. The amendment was adopted by voice vote.

2. Representative Suzanne Bonamici (D–OR) offered an amendment that adds a rule of construction that nothing prevents institutions of higher education from providing medically accurate and comprehensive information about abortion services. The amendment failed by a recorded vote of 15–23.

3. Representative Bob Good (R–VA) offered an amendment that adds data to the findings section of the bill on the impact of abortion on women's mental and physical health. The amendment was adopted by a recorded vote of 23–17.

1. Representative Kathy Manning (D–NC) offered an amendment that adds a rule of construction that nothing prevents an institution of higher education from providing medically accurate and comprehensive information about sexual and reproductive health services, including contraception. The amendment failed by a recorded vote of 17–23.

2. Representative Pramila Jayapal (D–WA) offered an amendment that requires institutions of higher education to also disseminate information on access to the Medicaid program, the supplemental nutrition assistance program (SNAP), and programs under Title X of the Public Health Services Act. The amendment failed by a recorded vote of 17–24.

3. Representative Haley Stevens (D–MI) offered an amendment that adds a rule of construction that nothing prevents an institution of higher education from disseminating information on resources (including available rights, protections and accommodations afforded to students under Title IX) regarding pregnancy and related medical conditions, including miscarriage. This amendment failed by a recorded vote of 17–24.

4. Representative Jahana Hayes (D–CT) offered an amendment that would incorporate the text of the American Family Act which creates a new program for the refundable child tax credit. This amendment was withdrawn.

Committee Views

Introduction

Pregnancy should not discourage a student from completing her education. Federal law prohibits discrimination against pregnant students and many resources are available to help expectant mothers through childbirth and parenting in college. Despite this, pregnant students are too often unaware of the rights and resources available to them, negatively impacting their ability to navigate options for balancing college and pregnancy. The Pregnant

Students Rights' Act aims to empower pregnant women to choose the best future for themselves and their child by having this information more easily accessible.

Mothers in Postsecondary Education

Today, policies at every level of government have enabled almost unfettered access to postsecondary education for many aspiring students. With increased access, 30 percent of enrolled students are now considered non-traditional students, meaning they are older, enrolled part-time, work full-time, or are financially independent but supporting dependents.[1] Student parents are a core component of the postsecondary education student body, as over 20 percent of all undergraduate students are parents.[2] Of these student parents, 43 percent are single mothers.[3] Overall, 10 percent, or 1.7 million, of all undergraduate students are single mothers, many of whom may no longer face access barriers to a college education but face uphill challenges when completing their education compared to women in college who are not mothers.[4] However, even with additional obstacles, such as more frequent absences from class, that often hinder their ability to graduate on time, student parents maintain higher grade point averages than other students.[5] This shows that student mothers are dedicated to excelling in their academic pursuits.

Title IX

Congress has acknowledged the importance of protecting equal access to postsecondary education for pregnant students. Title IX of the Education Amendments of 1972 (Title IX) prohibits recipients of federal funds from discriminating against students on the basis of sex.[6] Longstanding Title IX regulations from the Department of Education (Department) explicitly prohibit discrimination against pregnant women and the exclusion of pregnant

---

[1] https://pnpi.org/wp-content/uploads/2023/03/PostTraditional_FactSheet_Mar2023.pdf.

[2] https://iwpr.org/wp-content/uploads/2020/08/C481_Parents-in-College-By-the-Numbers-Aspen-Ascend-and-IWPR.pdf.

[3] *Ibid.*

[4] https://iwpr.org/wp-content/uploads/2020/07/R600_Investing-in-Single-Moms-National.pdf.

[5] https://iwpr.org/wp-content/uploads/2020/08/C481_Parents-in-College-By-the-Numbers-Aspen-Ascend-and-IWPR.pdf.

[6] Title IX of the Education Amendments of 1972.

women from an institution's education program because of pregnancy.[7] A student's rights under Title IX allow for protections and accommodations both in and out of the classroom, including the ability to take medically necessary leave and excused absences for pregnancy, childbirth, or related conditions.[8] Pregnant students are also protected from discrimination in institution-sponsored extracurricular activities, including internships, athletics, financial aid and scholarships, career counseling, and lab and clinical work.[9] Accommodations available to a pregnant student must be at least the same accommodations available to another student that has a temporary condition.

These robust protections for a woman's education during pregnancy allow her to successfully carry a baby to term without much additional worry about the impact on her education. However, almost 30 percent of all abortions in the United States are performed on women of college age, between the ages of 20 and 24, according to a 2021 report by the Centers for Disease Control and Prevention. Pregnant students should never feel obligated to seek an abortion to continue their education, but there are instances where students describe this type of pressure.[10]

Title IX also includes explicit statutory language regarding abortion that was added to the statute in 1988 and states, "Nothing in this title shall be construed to require or prohibit any person, or public or private entity, to provide or pay for any benefit or service, including the use of facilities, related to an abortion."[11] The intent of this language is to ensure that recipients of federal funds cannot be required to provide or pay for an abortion or abortion-related service under Title IX or be charged with violating Title IX if they choose to provide or pay for an abortion or abortion-related service. Depending on the pregnancy, a student may also be covered by disability protections and services under the Americans with Disabilities Act. A postsecondary institution must also provide a Title IX complaint process for when a student believes their Title IX rights have been violated. These current protections and accommodations for pregnant students can be utilized to ensure a pregnant student has the same opportunity to continue her education as any other student.

---

[7] 34 CFR 106.
[8] https://thepregnantscholar.org/title-ix-basics/.
[9] *Ibid.*
[10] https://www.foxnews.com/us/pro-life-group-mom-college-pregnant-parenting-rights.
[11] *Education Amendments of 1972*, § 909.

Lack of Awareness

While pregnant students' rights to postsecondary education exist, many students may be unaware of these rights or lack full information about possible accommodations or how to file a complaint. There are still instances in which students are advised to drop out because of their pregnancy, despite being allowed reasonable accommodation. In 2022, the Department's Office for Civil Rights determined that Salt Lake Community College violated both Title IX and Section 504 of the Rehabilitation Act of 1973 after a professor encouraged a pregnant student to drop a course because of ongoing absences due to her pregnancy.[12] The student had also informed the college's disability resource center and Title IX coordinator because she knew she was entitled to course modifications, but the college did not offer alternatives and the Title IX coordinator did not create an investigation file to look into the professor's actions. Additionally, in the Department's findings, the college's Code of Student Rights and Responsibilities did not provide information about the rights of pregnant students.[13] Transparent information is needed to ensure students know their rights and can navigate Title IX complaint and other campus processes. It is also needed to serve as an accountability mechanism for colleges and universities to not ignore their responsibility to provide these rights and accommodations.

Resources

There are many resources for pregnant students both on and off campus. These resources include between 2,600 and 2,700 pregnancy resource centers across the country in communities of all sizes. Pregnancy resource centers offer classes focused on the skills a pregnant mother may need and often serve as a place where mothers can receive basic baby items like diapers, formula, and clothing at no cost.[14]

---

[12] https://www.ed.gov/news/press-releases/us-department-educations-office-civil-rights- an nounces-resolution-pregnancy-discrimination-investigation-salt-lake-community-college.

[13] https://www.bsk.com/news-events-videos/office-for-civil-rights-faults-college-for-failing-to-accommodate-a-pregnant-student.

[14] https://www.focusonthefamily.com/pro-life/alternatives-to-abortion-pregnancy-resource- ce nters/.

Postsecondary education students are often already making a sacrifice of their time and finances in paying for college and an unplanned pregnancy can mean a pregnant student may need to draw upon even more outside resources. An estimated 12 percent of college students report experiencing an unplanned pregnancy.[15] There are other organizations that serve pregnant students, and some institutions are also focusing on reducing the stigma of unplanned pregnancy and creating a family-friendly campus environment.[16] A program known as Baby Steps at Auburn University serves both campus residents and community moms by providing housing, meals, access to pediatric care, counseling, academic advising, and tutoring, as well as by providing more information to students on education scholarships.[17] Belmont Abbey College hosts MiraVia, an on-campus maternity home that gives expectant mothers a place to live and care for their baby. Mothers at MiraVia work with staff to set goals for their education and future independence after they graduate. Belmont Abbey College allows pregnant mothers at MiraVia to enroll tuition-free.[18] Additionally, in Wyoming, the Adopt-a-College-Student program has developed a relationship with a local community college and the University of Wyoming to pair pregnant students with sponsors who provide mentorship and help with educational expenses.[19] These examples of partnerships to support pregnant mothers have been integral in furthering each parent's academic career.

Information Disclosure in Postsecondary Education

Section 485 of the Higher Education Act requires colleges and universities that receive Title IV funding to provide information on a variety of topics to prospective and enrolled students. This section of the law initially focused on disseminating information on the student financial assistance programs available to students but also requires institutions to disclose information about academic programs, costs of attending an institution, accreditation or licensing of an institution, standards for making satisfactory academic

---

[15] https://vtechworks.lib.vt.edu/items/747550b6-c0a8-4e66-b6d3-7f9c29e08596.

[16] https://www.npr.org/2019/05/02/716123170/do-they-kick-out-pregnant-people-navigating-college-with-kids.

[17] https://erlc.com/resource-library/articles/the-need-to-serve-pregnant-women-on-college- campuses/.

[18] https://www.liveaction.org/news/campus-maternity-home-support-pregnant/.

[19] https://pregnancyhelpnews.com/mommies-can-graduate-adopt-a-college-student-programs - help-pregnant-women-attend-college.

progress, and completion or graduation rates of an institution. Section 485 also requires institutions to provide disclosures through entrance and exit counseling to borrowers, disclosures on the number of students on athletically related student aid, transfer credit policies, fire safety standards, missing persons procedures, penalties for drug violations, and disclosures of campus crime statistics. This section ensures students have complete information on the costs and characteristics of the education an institution provides, as well as topics that affect campus life and may be adjacent to helping the student complete his or her education. Pregnant students' rights should be more publicly available as this growing student population seeks to obtain postsecondary education.

Conclusion

Students cannot assert their rights or seek helpful accommodations if these rights are not known. By ensuring pregnant students have information on available rights, accommodations, and resources, the Pregnant Students' Rights Act will ensure that all collegiate women are equipped with beneficial information to guide them on their path to becoming a mother and a graduate.

Summary

The Pregnant Students' Rights Act (H.R. 6914), introduced by Representative Hinson, would, as a condition of receiving Title IV funding, require colleges and universities to disseminate information to prospective and enrolled students on the rights of, and resources for, pregnant students and students who may become preg nant to carry a baby to term. The required information is a list of on-campus and community resources and accommodations available to help a pregnant student carry a baby to term and care for the baby after birth. The bill also requires institutions to disclose information on how to file a Title IX complaint with the Department or with the institution if a student believes that her Title IX rights were violated on account of her determination to carry a baby to term. The bill specifies that the required information dissemination must include an email to enrolled students at the start of each period of study during an academic year and the information to appear in student handbooks, at each orientation, at student health or counseling centers, as well as on the institution's website. A rule of construction clarifies that nothing in the new subsection created by this bill shall be construed to authorize the Secretary to require the dissemination of additional information, or establish additional rights, beyond the information and rights included in the subsection.

H.R. 6914 Section-by-Section Summary

Section 1. Short title

The short title is "Pregnant Students' Rights Act."

Section 2. Findings

This section describes the challenges pregnant college students may face when experiencing an unplanned pregnancy, including pressure to receive an abortion or lack of accommodations, which ultimately have a negative impact on the student's ability to continue her education.

Section 3. Notice of pregnant students' rights, accommodations, and resources

As a condition of receiving Title IV funding, this section requires colleges and universities to disseminate information to prospective and enrolled students on the rights of, and resources for, pregnant students and students who may become pregnant to carry a baby to term. The required information is a list of on-campus and community resources and accommodations available to help a pregnant student carry a baby to term and care for the baby after birth. This section also requires institutions to also disclose information on how to file a Title IX complaint with the Department or with the institution if a student believes that her Title IX rights were violated on account of her determination to carry a baby to term. The section specifies that the required information dissemination must include an email to enrolled students at the start of each period of study during an academic year and the information to appear in student handbooks, at each orientation, at student health or counseling centers, as well as on the institution's website. A rule of construction clarifies that nothing in the new subsection created by this bill shall be construed to authorize the Secretary to require the dissemination of additional information, or establish additional rights, beyond the information and rights included in the subsection.

Explanation of Amendments

The amendments, including the amendment in the nature of a substitute, are explained in the body of this report.

Application of Law to the Legislative Branch

Section 102(b)3 of Public Law 104–1 requires a description of the application of this bill to the Legislative Branch. H.R. 6914 requires institutions of higher education to disseminate information on the rights to, and accommodations and resources for, pregnant students to carry a baby to term. H.R. 6914 is applicable to institutions of higher education and therefore does not apply to the Legislative Branch.

Earmark Statement

H.R. 6914 does not contain any congressional earmarks, limited tax benefits, or limited tariff benefits as defined in clause 9 of rule XXI of the Rules of the House of Representatives.

Unfunded Mandate Statement

Pursuant to Section 423 of the Congressional Budget and Impoundment Control Act (as amended by Section 101(a)(2) of the Unfunded Mandates Reform Act, P.L. 104–4) the Committee adopts as its own the cost estimate prepared by the Congressional Budget Office (CBO) pursuant to section 402 of the Congressional Budget and Impoundment Control Act of 1974.

Roll Call Votes

Clause 3(b) of rule XIII of the Rules of the House of Representatives requires the Committee Report to include for each record vote on a motion to report the measure or matter and on any amendments offered to the measure or matter the total number of votes for and against and the names of the Members voting for and against.

Date: 1/10/24

COMMITTEE ON EDUCATION AND THE WORKFORCE RECORD OF COMMITTEE VOTE

Roll Call: 1 Bill: H.R. 6914 Amendment Number: n/a

Disposition: Not adopted by a Full Committee Roll Call Vote (15 y -23 n)

Sponsor/Amendment: Rep. Bonamici / AMD_01

Name & State	Aye	No	Not Voting	Name & State	Aye	No	Not Voting
Mrs. FOXX (NC) (Chairwoman)		X		Mr. SCOTT (VA) (Ranking)	X		
Mr. WILSON (SC)		X		Mr. GRIJALVA (AZ)	X		
Mr. THOMPSON (PA)		X		Mr. COURNTEY (CT)	X		
Mr. WALBERG (MI)		X		Mr. SABLAN (MP)	X		
Mr. GROTHMAN (WI)		X		Ms. WILSON (FL)			X
Ms. STEFANIK (NY)		X		Ms. BONAMICI (OR)	X		
Mr. ALLEN (GA)		X		Mr. TAKANO (CA)	X		
Mr. BANKS (IN)		X		Ms. ADAMS (NC)	X		
Mr. COMER (KY)			X	Mr. DESAULNIER (CA)	X		
Mr. SMUCKER (PA)			X	Mr. NORCROSS (NJ)	X		
Mr. OWENS (UT)		X		Ms. JAYAPAL (WA)	X		
Mr. GOOD (VA)		X		Ms. WILD (PA)			X
Mrs. MCCLAIN (MI)		X		Ms. MCBATH (GA)			X
Mrs. MILLER (IL)		X		Mrs. HAYES (CT)	X		
Mrs. STEEL (CA)		X		Ms. OMAR (MN)			X
Mr. ESTES (KS)		X		Ms. STEVENS (MI)	X		
Ms. LETLOW (LA)		X		Ms. LEGER FERNÁNDEZ (NM)	X		
Mr. KILEY (CA)		X		Ms. MANNING (NC)	X		
Mr. BEAN (FL)		X		Mr. MRVAN (IN)	X		
Mr. BURLISON (MO)		X		Mr. BOWMAN (NY)			X
Mr. MORAN (TX)		X					
Mr. JAMES (MI)		X					
Ms. CHAVEZ-DEREMER (OR)		X					
Mr. WILLIAMS (NY)		X					
Ms. HOUCHIN (IN)		X					

TOTALS: Ayes: 15 Nos: 23 Not Voting:7

Total: 45 / Quorum: 38/ Report:

(25 R - 20 D)

Date: 1/10/24

COMMITTEE ON EDUCATION AND THE WORKFORCE RECORD OF COMMITTEE VOTE

Roll Call: 2 Bill: H.R. 6914 Amendment Number: n/a

Disposition: Adopted by a Full Committee Roll Call Vote (23 y – 17 n)

Sponsor/Amendment: Rep. Good / GOOD_125

Name & State	Aye	No	Not Voting	Name & State	Aye	No	Not Voting
Mrs. FOXX (NC) (Chairwoman)	X			Mr. SCOTT (VA) (Ranking)		X	
Mr. WILSON (SC)	X			Mr. GRIJALVA (AZ)		X	
Mr. THOMPSON (PA)	X			Mr. COURNTEY (CT)		X	
Mr. WALBERG (MI)	X			Mr. SABLAN (MP)		X	
Mr. GROTHMAN (WI)	X			Ms. WILSON (FL)			X
Ms. STEFANIK (NY)	X			Ms. BONAMICI (OR)		X	
Mr. ALLEN (GA)	X			Mr. TAKANO (CA)		X	
Mr. BANKS (IN)	X			Ms. ADAMS (NC)		X	
Mr. COMER (KY)			X	Mr. DESAULNIER (CA)		X	
Mr. SMUCKER (PA)	X			Mr. NORCROSS (NJ)		X	
Mr. OWENS (UT)	X			Ms. JAYAPAL (WA)		X	
Mr. GOOD (VA)	X			Ms. WILD (PA)			X
Mrs. MCCLAIN (MI)	X			Ms. MCBATH (GA)			X
Mrs. MILLER (IL)	X			Mrs. HAYES (CT)		X	
Mrs. STEEL (CA)	X			Ms. OMAR (MN)		X	
Mr. ESTES (KS)	X			Ms. STEVENS (MI)		X	
Ms. LETLOW (LA)	X			Ms. LEGER FERNÁNDEZ (NM)		X	
Mr. KILEY (CA)	X			Ms. MANNING (NC)		X	
Mr. BEAN (FL)	X			Mr. MRVAN (IN)		X	
Mr. BURLISON (MO)	X			Mr. BOWMAN (NY)			X
Mr. MORAN (TX)	X						
Mr. JAMES (MI)	X						
Ms. CHAVEZ-DEREMER (OR)		X					
Mr. WILLIAMS (NY)	X						
Ms. HOUCHIN (IN)	X						

TOTALS: Ayes: 23 Nos: 17 Not Voting:5

Total: 45 / Quorum: 40/ Report:

(25 R - 20 D)

Date: 1/10/24

COMMITTEE ON EDUCATION AND THE WORKFORCE RECORD OF COMMITTEE VOTE

Roll Call: 3 Bill: H.R. 6914 Amendment Number: n/a

Disposition: Not adopted by a Full Committee Roll Call Vote (17 y – 23 n)

Sponsor/Amendment: Rep. Manning / AMD_02

Name & State	Aye	No	Not Voting	Name & State	Aye	No	Not Voting
Mrs. FOXX (NC) (Chairwoman)		X		Mr. SCOTT (VA) (Ranking)	X		
Mr. WILSON (SC)		X		Mr. GRIJALVA (AZ)	X		
Mr. THOMPSON (PA)		X		Mr. COURNTEY (CT)	X		
Mr. WALBERG (MI)		X		Mr. SABLAN (MP)	X		
Mr. GROTHMAN (WI)		X		Ms. WILSON (FL)			X
Ms. STEFANIK (NY)		X		Ms. BONAMICI (OR)	X		
Mr. ALLEN (GA)		X		Mr. TAKANO (CA)	X		
Mr. BANKS (IN)		X		Ms. ADAMS (NC)	X		
Mr. COMER (KY)			X	Mr. DESAULNIER (CA)	X		
Mr. SMUCKER (PA)		X		Mr. NORCROSS (NJ)	X		
Mr. OWENS (UT)		X		Ms. JAYAPAL (WA)	X		
Mr. GOOD (VA)		X		Ms. WILD (PA)			X
Mrs. MCCLAIN (MI)		X		Ms. MCBATH (GA)			X
Mrs. MILLER (IL)		X		Mrs. HAYES (CT)	X		
Mrs. STEEL (CA)		X		Ms. OMAR (MN)	X		
Mr. ESTES (KS)		X		Ms. STEVENS (MI)	X		
Ms. LETLOW (LA)		X		Ms. LEGER FERNÁNDEZ (NM)	X		
Mr. KILEY (CA)		X		Ms. MANNING (NC)	X		
Mr. BEAN (FL)		X		Mr. MRVAN (IN)	X		
Mr. BURLISON (MO)		X		Mr. BOWMAN (NY)			X
Mr. MORAN (TX)		X					
Mr. JAMES (MI)		X					
Ms. CHAVEZ-DEREMER (OR)	X						
Mr. WILLIAMS (NY)		X					
Ms. HOUCHIN (IN)		X					

TOTALS: Ayes: 17 Nos: 23 Not Voting: 5

Total: 45 / Quorum: 40/ Report:

(25 R - 20 D)

Date: 1/10/24

COMMITTEE ON EDUCATION AND THE WORKFORCE RECORD OF COMMITTEE VOTE

Roll Call: 4 Bill: H.R. 6914 Amendment Number: n/a

Disposition: Not Adopted by a Full Committee Roll Call Vote (17 y – 24 n)

Sponsor/Amendment: Rep. Jayapal / AMD_04

Name & State	Aye	No	Not Voting	Name & State	Aye	No	Not Voting
Mrs. FOXX (NC) (Chairwoman)		X		Mr. SCOTT (VA) (Ranking)	X		
Mr. WILSON (SC)		X		Mr. GRIJALVA (AZ)	X		
Mr. THOMPSON (PA)		X		Mr. COURNTEY (CT)	X		
Mr. WALBERG (MI)		X		Mr. SABLAN (MP)	X		
Mr. GROTHMAN (WI)		X		Ms. WILSON (FL)			X
Ms. STEFANIK (NY)		X		Ms. BONAMICI (OR)	X		
Mr. ALLEN (GA)		X		Mr. TAKANO (CA)	X		
Mr. BANKS (IN)		X		Ms. ADAMS (NC)	X		
Mr. COMER (KY)			X	Mr. DESAULNIER (CA)	X		
Mr. SMUCKER (PA)		X		Mr. NORCROSS (NJ)	X		
Mr. OWENS (UT)		X		Ms. JAYAPAL (WA)	X		
Mr. GOOD (VA)		X		Ms. WILD (PA)	X		
Mrs. MCCLAIN (MI)		X		Ms. MCBATH (GA)			X
Mrs. MILLER (IL)		X		Mrs. HAYES (CT)	X		
Mrs. STEEL (CA)		X		Ms. OMAR (MN)	X		
Mr. ESTES (KS)		X		Ms. STEVENS (MI)	X		
Ms. LETLOW (LA)		X		Ms. LEGER FERNÁNDEZ (NM)	X		
Mr. KILEY (CA)		X		Ms. MANNING (NC)	X		
Mr. BEAN (FL)		X		Mr. MRVAN (IN)	X		
Mr. BURLISON (MO)		X		Mr. BOWMAN (NY)			X
Mr. MORAN (TX)		X					
Mr. JAMES (MI)		X					
Ms. CHAVEZ-DEREMER (OR)		X					
Mr. WILLIAMS (NY)		X					
Ms. HOUCHIN (IN)		X					

TOTALS: Ayes: 17 Nos: 24 Not Voting: 4

Total: 45 / Quorum: 41 / Report:

(25 R - 20 D)

Date: 1/10/24

COMMITTEE ON EDUCATION AND THE WORKFORCE RECORD OF COMMITTEE VOTE

Roll Call: 5 Bill: H.R. 6914 Amendment Number: n/a

Disposition: Not Adopted by a Full Committee Roll Call Vote (17 y – 24 n)

Sponsor/Amendment: Rep. Stevens / AMD_05

Name & State	Aye	No	Not Voting	Name & State	Aye	No	Not Voting
Mrs. FOXX (NC) (Chairwoman)		X		Mr. SCOTT (VA) (Ranking)	X		
Mr. WILSON (SC)		X		Mr. GRIJALVA (AZ)	X		
Mr. THOMPSON (PA)		X		Mr. COURNTEY (CT)	X		
Mr. WALBERG (MI)		X		Mr. SABLAN (MP)	X		
Mr. GROTHMAN (WI)		X		Ms. WILSON (FL)			X
Ms. STEFANIK (NY)		X		Ms. BONAMICI (OR)	X		
Mr. ALLEN (GA)		X		Mr. TAKANO (CA)	X		
Mr. BANKS (IN)		X		Ms. ADAMS (NC)	X		
Mr. COMER (KY)			X	Mr. DESAULNIER (CA)	X		
Mr. SMUCKER (PA)		X		Mr. NORCROSS (NJ)	X		
Mr. OWENS (UT)		X		Ms. JAYAPAL (WA)	X		
Mr. GOOD (VA)		X		Ms. WILD (PA)	X		
Mrs. MCCLAIN (MI)		X		Ms. MCBATH (GA)			X
Mrs. MILLER (IL)		X		Mrs. HAYES (CT)	X		
Mrs. STEEL (CA)		X		Ms. OMAR (MN)	X		
Mr. ESTES (KS)		X		Ms. STEVENS (MI)	X		
Ms. LETLOW (LA)		X		Ms. LEGER FERNÁNDEZ (NM)	X		
Mr. KILEY (CA)		X		Ms. MANNING (NC)	X		
Mr. BEAN (FL)		X		Mr. MRVAN (IN)	X		
Mr. BURLISON (MO)		X		Mr. BOWMAN (NY)			X
Mr. MORAN (TX)		X					
Mr. JAMES (MI)		X					
Ms. CHAVEZ-DEREMER (OR)		X					
Mr. WILLIAMS (NY)		X					
Ms. HOUCHIN (IN)		X					

TOTALS: Ayes: 17 Nos: 24 Not Voting:4

Total: 45 / Quorum:41 / Report:

(25 R - 20 D)

Date: 1/10/24

COMMITTEE ON EDUCATION AND THE WORKFORCE RECORD OF COMMITTEE VOTE

Roll Call: 6 Bill: H.R 6914 Amendment Number: n/a

Disposition: Adopted by a Full Committee Roll Call Vote (24 y -17 n)

Sponsor/Amendment: Rep. Miller / ANS_01 / Motion to Report

Name & State	Aye	No	Not Voting	Name & State	Aye	No	Not Voting
Mrs. FOXX (NC) (Chairwoman)	X			Mr. SCOTT (VA) (Ranking)		X	
Mr. WILSON (SC)	X			Mr. GRIJALVA (AZ)		X	
Mr. THOMPSON (PA)	X			Mr. COURNTEY (CT)		X	
Mr. WALBERG (MI)	X			Mr. SABLAN (MP)		X	
Mr. GROTHMAN (WI)	X			Ms. WILSON (FL)			X
Ms. STEFANIK (NY)	X			Ms. BONAMICI (OR)		X	
Mr. ALLEN (GA)	X			Mr. TAKANO (CA)		X	
Mr. BANKS (IN)	X			Ms. ADAMS (NC)		X	
Mr. COMER (KY)			X	Mr. DESAULNIER (CA)		X	
Mr. SMUCKER (PA)	X			Mr. NORCROSS (NJ)		X	
Mr. OWENS (UT)	X			Ms. JAYAPAL (WA)		X	
Mr. GOOD (VA)	X			Ms. WILD (PA)		X	
Mrs. MCCLAIN (MI)	X			Ms. MCBATH (GA)			X
Mrs. MILLER (IL)	X			Mrs. HAYES (CT)		X	
Mrs. STEEL (CA)	X			Ms. OMAR (MN)		X	
Mr. ESTES (KS)	X			Ms. STEVENS (MI)		X	
Ms. LETLOW (LA)	X			Ms. LEGER FERNÁNDEZ (NM)		X	
Mr. KILEY (CA)	X			Ms. MANNING (NC)		X	
Mr. BEAN (FL)	X			Mr. MRVAN (IN)		X	
Mr. BURLISON (MO)	X			Mr. BOWMAN (NY)			X
Mr. MORAN (TX)	X						
Mr. JAMES (MI)	X						
Ms. CHAVEZ-DEREMER (OR)	X						
Mr. WILLIAMS (NY)	X						
Ms. HOUCHIN (IN)	X						

TOTALS: Ayes: 24 Nos: 17 Not Voting: 4

Total: 45 / Quorum: 41/ Report:

(25 R - 20 D)

New Budget Authority and CBO Cost Estimate

With respect to the requirements of clause 3(c)(2) of rule XIII of the Rules of the House of Representatives and section 308(a) of the Congressional Budget Act of 1974 and with respect to requirements of clause 3(c)(3) of rule XIII of the Rules of the House of Representatives and section 402 of the Congressional Budget Act of 1974, the Committee has received the following estimate for H.R. 6914 from the Director of the Congressional Budget Office:

H.R. 6914, Pregnant Students' Rights Act
As ordered reported by the House Committee on Education and the Workforce on January 10, 2024

By Fiscal Year, Millions of Dollars	2024	2024-2028	2024-2033
Direct Spending (Outlays)	0	0	0
Revenues	0	0	0
Increase or Decrease (-) in the Deficit	0	0	0
Spending Subject to Appropriation (Outlays)	*	*	not estimated

Increases *net direct spending* in any of the four consecutive 10-year periods beginning in 2034?	No	Statutory pay-as-you-go procedures apply?	No
		Mandate Effects	
Increases *on-budget deficits* in any of the four consecutive 10-year periods beginning in 2034?	No	Contains intergovernmental mandate?	No
		Contains private-sector mandate?	No

* = between zero and $500,000.

H.R. 6914 would require institutions of higher education that receive federal student aid under title IV of the Higher Education Act to provide specific information on the rights of pregnant students. Those requirements include a list of on-campus and community resources that exist to help pregnant students carry a baby to term, information about accommodations available to students during and after pregnancy, and information on how to report a violation of those rights.

CBO expects that institutions would comply with the requirements in the bill to remain eligible for federal student aid. As a result, CBO estimates enacting the bill would have no effect on federal spending for student aid.

Based on the cost of similar activities, CBO estimates that the Department of Education's cost to implement H.R. 6914 would not be significant; any spending would be subject to the availability of appropriated funds.

The CBO staff contact for this estimate is Leah Koestner. The estimate was reviewed by H. Samuel Papenfuss, Deputy Director of Budget Analysis.

Phillip L. Swagel,
Director, Congressional Budget Office.

Committee Cost Estimate

Clause 3(d)(1) of rule XIII of the Rules of the House of Representatives requires an estimate and a comparison of the costs that would be incurred in carrying out H.R. 6914. However, clause 3(d)(2)(B) of that rule provides that this requirement does not apply when, as with the present report, the Committee adopts as its own the cost estimate of the bill prepared by the Director of the Congressional Budget Office under section 402 of the Congressional Budget Act.

Statement of General Performance Goals and Objectives

In accordance with clause (3)(c) of rule XIII of the Rules of the House of Representatives, the goal of H.R. 6914 is to ensure pregnant students attending institutions of higher education receive information on the rights of, and accommodations and resources for, pregnant students.

Duplication of Federal Programs

No provision of H.R. 6914 establishes or reauthorizes a program of the Federal Government known to be duplicative of another Federal program, a program that was included in any report from the Government Accountability Office to Congress pursuant to section 21 of Public Law 111–139, or a program related to a program identified in the most recent Catalog of Federal Domestic Assistance.

Statement of Oversight Findings and Recommendations of the Committee

In compliance with clause 3(c)(1) of rule XIII and clause 2(b)(1) of rule X of the Rules of the House of Representatives, the committee's oversight findings and recommendations are reflected in the body of this report.

Required Committee Hearing and Related Hearings

In compliance with clause 3(c)(6) of rule XIII of the Rules of the House of Representatives the following hearings held during the 118th Congress were used to develop or consider H.R. 6914: On May 16, 2023, the Committee on Education and the Workforce held a hearing on "Examining the Policies and Priorities of the U.S. Department of Education"; on June 14, 2023, the Subcommittee on Higher Education and Workforce Development held a hearing on "Postsecondary Innovation: Preparing Today's Students For Tomorrow's Opportunities."

Changes in Existing Law Made by the Bill, as Reported

In compliance with clause 3(e) of rule XIII of the Rules of the House of Representatives, changes in existing law made by the bill, as reported, are shown as follows (new matter is printed in italics and existing law in which no change is proposed is shown in roman):

Higher Education Act of 1965

* * * * * *

* TITLE IV—STUDENT ASSISTANCE

* * * * * * *

PART G—GENERAL PROVISIONS RELATING TO STUDENT ASSISTANCE PROGRAMS

* * * * * * *

SEC. 485. INSTITUTIONAL AND FINANCIAL ASSISTANCE INFORMATION FOR STUDENTS.

(a) INFORMATION DISSEMINATION ACTIVITIES.— (1) Each eligible institution participating in any program under this title shall carry out information dissemination activities for prospective and enrolled students (including those attending or planning to attend less than full time) regarding the institution and all financial assistance under this title. The information required by this section shall be produced and be made readily available upon request, through appropriate publications, mailings, and electronic media, to an enrolled student and to any prospective student. Each eligible institution shall, on an annual basis, provide to all enrolled students a list of the information that is required to be provided by institutions to students by this section and section 444 of the General Education Provisions Act (commonly known as the "Family Educational Rights and Privacy Act of 1974"), together with a statement of the procedures required to obtain such information. The information required by this section shall accurately describe—

(A) the student financial assistance programs available to students who enroll at such institution;

(B) the methods by which such assistance is distributed among student recipients who enroll at such institution;

(C) any means, including forms, by which application for student financial assistance is made and requirements for accurately preparing such application;

(D) the rights and responsibilities of students receiving financial assistance under this title;

(E) the cost of attending the institution, including (i) tuition and fees, (ii) books and supplies, (iii) estimates of typical student room and board costs or typical commuting costs, and (iv) any additional cost of the program in which the student is enrolled or expresses a specific interest;

(F) a statement of—

(i) the requirements of any refund policy with which the institution is required to comply;

(ii) the requirements under section 484B for the return of grant or loan assistance provided under this title; and

(iii) the requirements for officially withdrawing from the institution;

(G) the academic program of the institution, including (i) the current degree programs and other educational and training programs, (ii) the instructional, laboratory, and other physical plant facilities which relate to the academic program, (iii) the faculty and other instructional personnel, and (iv) any plans by the institution for improving the academic program of the institution;

(H) each person designated under subsection (c) of this section, and the methods by which and locations in which any person so designated may be contacted by students and prospective students who are seeking information required by this subsection;

(I) special facilities and services available to students with disabilities;

(J) the names of associations, agencies, or governmental bodies which accredit, approve, or license the institution and its programs, and the procedures under which any current or prospective student may obtain or review upon request a copy of the documents describing the institution's accreditation, approval, or licensing;

(K) the standards which the student must maintain in order to be considered to be making satisfactory progress, pursuant to section 484(a)(2);

(L) the completion or graduation rate of certificate- or degree-seeking, full-time, undergraduate students entering such institutions;

(M) the terms and conditions of the loans that students receive under parts B, D, and E;

(N) that enrollment in a program of study abroad approved for credit by the home institution may be considered enrollment in the home institution for purposes of applying for Federal student financial assistance;

(O) the campus crime report prepared by the institution pursuant to subsection (f), including all required reporting categories;

(P) institutional policies and sanctions related to copyright infringement, including—

(i) an annual disclosure that explicitly informs students that unauthorized distribution of copyrighted material, including unauthorized peer-to-peer file sharing, may subject the students to civil and criminal liabilities;

(ii) a summary of the penalties for violation of Federal copyright laws; and

(iii) a description of the institution's policies with respect to unauthorized peer-to-peer file sharing, including disciplinary actions that are taken against students who engage in unauthorized distribution of copyrighted materials using the institution's information technology system;

(Q) student body diversity at the institution, including information on the percentage of enrolled, full-time students who—

(i) are male;

(ii) are female;

(iii) receive a Federal Pell Grant; and

(iv) are a self-identified member of a major racial or ethnic group;

(R) the placement in employment of, and types of employment obtained by, graduates of the institution's degree or certificate programs, gathered from such sources as alumni surveys, student satisfaction surveys, the National Survey of Student Engagement, the Community College Survey of Student Engagement, State data systems, or other relevant sources;

(S) the types of graduate and professional education in which graduates of the institution's four-year degree pro grams enrolled, gathered from such sources as alumni surveys, student satisfaction surveys, the National Survey of Student Engagement, State data systems, or other relevant sources;

(T) the fire safety report prepared by the institution pursuant to subsection (i);

(U) the retention rate of certificate- or degree-seeking, first-time, full-time, undergraduate students entering such institution; and

(V) institutional policies regarding vaccinations.

(2) For the purpose of this section, the term "prospective student" means any individual who has contacted an eligible institution requesting information concerning admission to that institution.

(3) In calculating the completion or graduation rate under sub-paragraph (L) of paragraph (1) of this subsection or under sub-section (e), a student shall be counted as a completion or graduation if, within 150 percent of the normal time for completion of or graduation from the program, the student has completed or graduated from the program, or enrolled in any program of an eligible institution for which the prior program provides substantial preparation. The information required to be disclosed under such subparagraph—

(A) shall be made available by July 1 each year to enrolled students and prospective students prior to the students enrolling or entering into any financial obligation; and

(B) shall cover the one-year period ending on August 31 of the preceding year.

(4) For purposes of this section, institutions may—

(A) exclude from the information disclosed in accordance with subparagraph (L) of paragraph (1) the completion or graduation rates of students who leave school to serve in the Armed Forces, on official church missions, or with a recognized foreign aid service of the Federal Government; or

(B) in cases where the students described in subparagraph (A) represent 20 percent or more of the certificate- or degree-seeking, full-time, undergraduate students at the institution, recalculate the completion or graduation rates of such students by excluding from the calculation described in paragraph (3) the time period during which such students were not enrolled due to their service in the Armed Forces, on official church missions, or with a recognized foreign aid service of the Federal Government.

(5) The Secretary shall permit any institution of higher education that is a member of an athletic association or athletic conference that has voluntarily published completion or graduation rate data or has agreed to publish data that, in the opinion of the Secretary, is substantially comparable to the information required under this subsection, to use such data to satisfy the requirements of this subsection; and

(6) Each institution may provide supplemental information to enrolled and prospective students showing the completion or graduation rate for students described in paragraph (4) or for students transferring into the institution or information showing the rate at which students transfer out of the institution.

(7)(A)(i) Subject to clause (ii), the information disseminated under paragraph (1)(L), or reported under subsection (e), shall be disaggregated by gender, by each major racial and ethnic subgroup, by recipients of a Federal Pell Grant, by recipients of a loan made under part B or D (other than a loan made under section 428H or a Federal Direct Unsubsidized Stafford Loan) who did not receive a Federal Pell Grant, and by recipients of neither a Federal Pell Grant nor a loan made under part B or D (other than a loan made under section 428H or a Federal Direct Unsubsidized Stafford Loan), if the number of students in such subgroup or with such status is sufficient to yield statistically reliable information and reporting will not reveal personally identifiable information about an individual student. If such number is not sufficient for such purposes, then the institution shall note that the institution enrolled too few of such students to so disclose or report with confidence and confidentiality.

(ii) The requirements of clause (i) shall not apply to two- year, degree-granting institutions of higher education until academic year 2011-2012.

(B)(i) In order to assist two-year degree-granting institutions of higher education in meeting the requirements of paragraph (1)(L) and subsection (e), the Secretary, in consultation with the Commissioner for Education Statistics, shall, not later than 90 days after the date of enactment of the Higher Education Opportunity Act, convene a group of representatives from diverse institutions of higher education, experts in the field of higher education policy, state higher education officials, students, and other stakeholders in the higher education community, to develop recommendations regarding the accurate calculation and reporting of the information required to be disseminated or reported under paragraph (1)(L) and subsection

(e) by two-year, degree-granting institutions of higher education. In developing such recommendations, the group of representatives shall consider the mission and role of two-year degree-granting institutions of higher education, and may recommend additional or alternative measures of student success for such institutions in light of the mission and role of such institutions.

(ii) The Secretary shall widely disseminate the recommendations required under this subparagraph to two-year, degree-granting institutions of higher education, the public, and the authorizing committees not later than 18 months after the first meeting of the group of representatives convened under clause (i).

(iii) The Secretary shall use the recommendations from the group of representatives convened under clause (i) to provide technical assistance to two-year, degree-granting institutions of higher education in meeting the requirements of paragraph (1)(L) and subsection (e).

(iv) The Secretary may modify the information required to be disseminated or reported under paragraph (1)(L) or subsection

(e) by a two-year, degree-granting institution of higher education—

(I) based on the recommendations received under this subparagraph from the group of representatives convened under clause (i);

(II) to include additional or alternative measures of student success if the goals of the provisions of paragraph (1)(L) and subsection (e) can be met through additional means or comparable alternatives; and

(III) during the period beginning on the date of enactment of the Higher Education Opportunity Act, and ending on June 30, 2011.

(a) EXIT COUNSELING FOR BORROWERS. — (1)(A) Each eligible institution shall, through financial aid offices or otherwise, provide counseling to borrowers of loans that are made, insured, or guaranteed under part B (other than loans made pursuant to section 428C or loans under section 428B made on behalf of a student) or made under part D (other than Federal Direct Consolidation Loans or Federal Direct PLUS Loans made on behalf of a student) or made under part E of this title prior to the completion of the course of study for which the borrower enrolled at the institution or at the time of departure from such institution. The counseling required by this subsection shall include—

(i) information on the repayment plans available, including a description of the different features of each plan and sample information showing the average anticipated monthly payments, and the difference in interest paid and total payments, under each plan;

(ii) debt management strategies that are designed to facilitate the repayment of such indebtedness;

(iii) an explanation that the borrower has the options to prepay each loan, pay each loan on a shorter schedule, and change repayment plans;

(iv) for any loan forgiveness or cancellation provision of this title, a general description of the terms and conditions under which the borrower may obtain full or partial forgiveness or cancellation of the principal and interest, and a copy of the information provided by the Secretary under section 485(d);

(V) for any forbearance provision of this title, a general description of the terms and conditions under which the borrower may defer repayment of principal or interest or be granted forbearance, and a copy of the information provided by the Secretary under section 485(d);

(vi) the consequences of defaulting on a loan, including adverse credit reports, delinquent debt collection procedures under Federal law, and litigation;

(vii) information on the effects of using a consolidation loan under section 428C or a Federal Direct Consolidation Loan to discharge the borrower's loans under parts B, D, and E, including at a minimum—

(I) the effects of consolidation on total interest to be paid, fees to be paid, and length of repayment;

(II) the effects of consolidation on a borrower's underlying loan benefits, including grace periods, loan forgiveness, cancellation, and deferment opportunities;

(III) the option of the borrower to prepay the loan or to change repayment plans; and

(I) that borrower benefit programs may vary among different lenders;

(ii) a general description of the types of tax benefits that may be available to borrowers;

(iii) a notice to borrowers about the availability of the National Student Loan Data System and how the system can be used by a borrower to obtain information on the status of the borrower's loans; and an explanation that—

(I) the borrower may be contacted during the repayment period by third-party student debt relief companies;

(II) the borrower should use caution when dealing with those companies; and

(III) the services that those companies typically provide are already offered to borrowers free of charge through the Department or the borrower's servicer; and

(B) In the case of borrower who leaves an institution without the prior knowledge of the institution, the institution shall attempt to provide the information described in subparagraph (A) to the student in writing.

(2)(A) Each eligible institution shall require that the borrower of a loan made under part B, D, or E submit to the institution, during the exit interview required by this subsection—

(i) the borrower's expected permanent address after leaving the institution (regardless of the reason for leaving);

(ii) the name and address of the borrower's expected employer after leaving the institution;

(iii) the address of the borrower's next of kin; and

(iv) any corrections in the institution's records relating the borrower's name, address, social security number, references, and driver's license number.

(B) The institution shall, within 60 days after the interview, forward any corrected or completed information received from the borrower to the guaranty agency indicated on the borrower's student aid records.

(c) Nothing in this subsection shall be construed to prohibit an institution of higher education from utilizing electronic means to provide personalized exit counseling.

(a) FINANCIAL ASSISTANCE INFORMATION PERSONNEL.—Each eligible institution shall designate an employee or group of employees who shall be available on a full-time basis to assist students or potential students in obtaining information as specified in subsection

(a). The Secretary may, by regulation, waive the requirement that an employee or employees be available on a full-time basis for carrying out responsibilities required under this section whenever an institution in which the total enrollment, or the portion of the enrollment participating in programs under this title at that institution, is too small to necessitate such employee or employees being available on a full-time basis. No such waiver may include permission to exempt any such institution from designating a specific individual or a group of individuals to carry out the provisions of this section.

(b) DEPARTMENTAL PUBLICATION OF DESCRIPTIONS OF ASSISTANCE

PROGRAMS.—(1) The Secretary shall make available to eligible institutions, eligible lenders, and secondary schools descriptions of Federal student assistance programs including the rights and responsibilities of student and institutional participants, in order to

(A) assist students in gaining information through institutional sources, and (B) assist institutions in carrying out the provisions of this section, so that individual and institutional participants will be fully aware of their rights and responsibilities under such programs. In particular, such information shall include information to enable students and prospective students to assess the debt burden and monthly and total repayment obligations that will be incurred as a result of receiving loans of varying amounts under this title. Such information shall also include information on the various payment options available for student loans, including income-sensitive and income-based repayment plans for loans made, insured, or guaranteed under part B and income-contingent and income- based repayment plans for loans made under part D. In addition, such information shall include information to enable borrowers to assess the practical consequences of loan consolidation, including differences in deferment eligibility, interest rates, monthly payments, and finance charges, and samples of loan consolidation profiles to illustrate such consequences. The Secretary shall provide information concerning the specific terms and conditions under which students may obtain partial or total cancellation or defer repayment of loans for service, shall indicate (in terms of the Federal minimum wage) the maximum level of compensation and allowances that a student borrower may receive from a tax-exempt organization to qualify for a deferment, and shall explicitly state that students may qualify for such partial cancellations or deferments when they serve as a paid employee of a tax-exempt organization. The Secretary shall also provide information on loan forbearance, including the increase in debt that results from capitalization of interest. Such information shall be provided by eligible institutions and eligible lenders at any time that information regarding loan availability is provided to any student.

(2) The Secretary, to the extent the information is available, shall compile information describing State and other prepaid tuition programs and savings programs and disseminate such information to States, eligible institutions, students, and parents in departmental publications.

(3) The Secretary, to the extent practicable, shall update the Department's Internet site to include direct links to databases that contain information on public and private financial assistance programs. The Secretary shall only provide direct links to databases that can be accessed without charge and shall make reasonable efforts to verify that the databases included in a direct link are not providing fraudulent information. The Secretary shall prominently

display adjacent to any such direct link a disclaimer indicating that a direct link to a database does not constitute an endorsement or recommendation of the database, the provider of the database, or any services or products of such provider. The Secretary shall provide additional direct links to information resources from which students may obtain information about fraudulent and deceptivepractices in the provision of services related to student financial aid.

(3) The Secretary shall widely publicize the location of the information described in paragraph (1) among the public, eligible institutions, and eligible lenders, and promote the use of such information by prospective students, enrolled students, families of prospective and enrolled students, and borrowers.

(c) DISCLOSURES REQUIRED WITH RESPECT TO ATHLETICALLY RELATED STUDENT AID.—(1) Each institution of higher education which participates in any program under this title and is attended by students receiving athletically related student aid shall annually submit a report to the Secretary which contains—

(A) the number of students at the institution of higher education who received athletically related student aid broken down by race and sex in the following sports: basketball, football, baseball, cross country/track, and all other sports combined;

(B) the number of students at the institution of higher education, broken down by race and sex;

(C) the completion or graduation rate for students at the institution of higher education who received athletically related student aid broken down by race and sex in the following sports: basketball, football, baseball, cross country/track and all other sports combined;

(D) the completion or graduation rate for students at the institution of higher education, broken down by race and sex;

(E) the average completion or graduation rate for the 4 most recent completing or graduating classes of students at the institution of higher education who received athletically related student aid broken down by race and sex in the following categories: basketball, football, baseball, cross country/track, and all other sports combined; and

(F) the average completion or graduation rate for the 4 most recent completing or graduating classes of students at the institution of higher education broken down by race and sex.

(2) When an institution described in paragraph (1) of this subsection offers a potential student athlete athletically related student aid, such institution shall provide to the student and the student's parents, guidance counselor, and coach

the information contained in the report submitted by such institution pursuant to paragraph (1). If the institution is a member of a national collegiate athletic association that compiles graduation rate data on behalf of the association's member institutions that the Secretary determines is substantially comparable to the information described in paragraph (1), the distribution of the compilation of such data to all secondary schools in the United States shall fulfill the responsibility of the institution to provide information to a prospective student athlete's guidance counselor and coach.

(3) For purposes of this subsection, institutions may—exclude from the reporting requirements under paragraphs (1) and (2) the completion or graduation rates of students and student athletes who leave school to serve in the Armed Forces, on official church missions, or with a recognized foreign aid service of the Federal Government; or

(A) in cases where the students described in subparagraph (A) represent 20 percent or more of the certificate- or degree-seeking, full-time, undergraduate students at the institution, calculate the completion or graduation rates of such students by excluding from the calculations described in paragraph (1) the time period during which such students were not enrolled due to their service in the Armed Forces, on official church missions, or with a recognized foreign aid service of the Federal Government.

(4) Each institution of higher education described in paragraph

(1) may provide supplemental information to students and the Secretary showing the completion or graduation rate when such completion or graduation rate includes students transferring into and out of such institution.

(5) The Secretary, using the reports submitted under this subsection, shall compile and publish a report containing the information required under paragraph (1) broken down by—

(A) individual institutions of higher education; and

(B) athletic conferences recognized by the National Collegiate Athletic Association and the National Association of Intercolle- giate Athletics.

(6) The Secretary shall waive the requirements of this subsection for any institution of higher education that is a member of an athletic association or athletic conference that has voluntarily published completion or graduation rate data or has agreed to publish data that, in the opinion of the Secretary, is substantially comparable to the information required under this subsection.

(7) The Secretary, in conjunction with the National Junior College Athletic Association, shall develop and obtain data on completion or graduation rates from two-year colleges that award athletically related student

aid. Such data shall, to the extent practicable, be consistent with the reporting requirements set forth in this section.

(8) For purposes of this subsection, the term "athletically related student aid" means any scholarship, grant, or other form of financial assistance the terms of which require the recipient to participate in a program of intercollegiate athletics at an institution of higher education in order to be eligible to receive such assistance.

(9) The reports required by this subsection shall be due each July 1 and shall cover the 1-year period ending August 31 of the preceding year.

(d) DISCLOSURE OF CAMPUS SECURITY POLICY AND CAMPUS CRIME STATISTICS.—(1) Each eligible institution participating in any program under this title, other than a foreign institution of higher education, shall on August 1, 1991, begin to collect the following information with respect to campus crime statistics and campus security policies of that institution, and beginning September 1, 1992, and each year thereafter, prepare, publish, and distribute, through appropriate publications or mailings, to all current students and employees, and to any applicant for enrollment or employment upon request, an annual security report containing at least the following information with respect to the campus security policies and campus crime statistics of that institution:

(A) A statement of current campus policies regarding procedures and facilities for students and others to report criminal actions or other emergencies occurring on campus and policies concerning the institution's response to such reports.

(A) A statement of current policies concerning security and access to campus facilities, including campus residences, and security considerations used in the maintenance of campus facilities.

(B) A statement of current policies concerning campus law enforcement, including—

(i) the law enforcement authority of campus security personnel;

(ii) the working relationship of campus security personnel with State and local law enforcement agencies, including whether the institution has agreements with such agencies, such as written memoranda of understanding, for the investigation of alleged criminal offenses; and

(iii) policies which encourage accurate and prompt reporting of all crimes to the campus police and the appropriate law enforcement agencies, when the victim of such crime elects or is unable to make such a report.

(C) A description of the type and frequency of programs designed to inform students and employees about campus security procedures and practices and to encourage students and employees to be responsible for their own security and the security of others.

(D) A description of programs designed to inform students and employees about the prevention of crimes.

(E) Statistics concerning the occurrence on campus, in or on noncampus buildings or property, and on public property during the most recent calendar year, and during the 2 preceding calendar years for which data are available—

(i) of the following criminal offenses reported to campus security authorities or local police agencies:

(I) murder;

(II) sex offenses, forcible or nonforcible;

(III)robbery;

(IV) aggravated assault;

(V) burglary;

(VI) motor vehicle theft;

(VII) manslaughter;

(VIII) arson;

(IX) arrests or persons referred for campus disciplinary action for liquor law violations, drug-related violations, and weapons possession; and

(ii) of the crimes described in subclauses (I) through

(VIII) of clause (i), of larceny-theft, simple assault, intimidation, and destruction, damage, or vandalism of property, and of other crimes involving bodily injury to any person, in which the victim is intentionally selected because of the actual or perceived race, gender, religion, national origin, sexual orientation, gender identity, ethnicity, or disability of the victim that are reported to campus security authorities or local police agencies, which data shall be collected and reported according to category of prejudice; and

(iii) of domestic violence, dating violence, and stalking incidents that were reported to campus security authorities or local police agencies.

(F) A statement of policy concerning the monitoring and recording through local police agencies of criminal activity at off-campus student organizations which are recognized by the institution and that are engaged in by students attending the institution, including those student organizations with off-campus housing facilities.

(G) A statement of policy regarding the possession, use, and sale of alcoholic beverages and enforcement of State underage drinking laws and a statement of policy regarding the possession, use, and sale of illegal drugs and enforcement of Federal and State drug laws and a description of any drug or alcohol abuse education programs as required under section 120 of this Act.

(H) A statement advising the campus community where law enforcement agency information provided by a State under section 170101(j) of the Violent Crime Control and Law Enforcement Act of 1994 (42 U.S.C. 14071(j)), concerning registered sex offenders may be obtained, such as the law enforcement office of the institution, a local law enforcement agency with jurisdiction for the campus, or a computer network address.

(I) A statement of current campus policies regarding immediate emergency response and evacuation procedures, including the use of electronic and cellular communication (if appropriate), which policies shall include procedures to—

(i) immediately notify the campus community upon the confirmation of a significant emergency or dangerous situation involving an immediate threat to the health or safety of students or staff occurring on the campus, as defined in paragraph (6), unless issuing a notification will compromise efforts to contain the emergency;

(ii) publicize emergency response and evacuation procedures on an annual basis in a manner designed to reach students and staff; and

(iii) test emergency response and evacuation procedures on an annual basis.

(1) Nothing in this subsection shall be construed to authorize the Secretary to require particular policies, procedures, or practices by institutions of higher education with respect to campus crimes or campus security.

(2) Each institution participating in any program under this title, other than a foreign institution of higher education, shall make timely reports to the campus community on crimes considered to be a threat to other students and employees described in paragraph (1)(F) that are reported to campus security or local law police agencies. Such reports shall be provided to students and employees in a manner that is timely, that withholds the names of victims as confidential, and that will aid in the prevention of similar occurrences.

(4)(A) Each institution participating in any program under this title, other than a foreign institution of higher education, that maintains a police or security department of any kind shall make, keep, and maintain a daily log, written in a form that can be easily understood, recording all crimes reported to such police or security department, including—

(i) the nature, date, time, and general location of each crime; and

(ii) the disposition of the complaint, if known.

(B)(i) All entries that are required pursuant to this paragraph shall, except where disclosure of such information is prohibited by law or such disclosure would jeopardize the confidentiality of the victim, be open to public inspection within two business days of the initial report being made to the department or a campus security authority.

(ii) If new information about an entry into a log becomes available to a police or security department, then the new information shall be recorded in the log not later than two business days after the information becomes available to the police or security department.

(iii) If there is clear and convincing evidence that the release of such information would jeopardize an ongoing criminal investigation or the safety of an individual, cause a suspect to flee or evade detection, or result in the destruction of evidence, such information may be withheld until that damage is no longer likely to occur from the release of such information.

(2) On an annual basis, each institution participating in any program under this title, other than a foreign institution of higher education, shall submit to the Secretary a copy of the statistics required to be made available under paragraph (1)(F). The Secretary shall—

(A) review such statistics and report to the authorizing committees on campus crime statistics by September 1, 2000;

(B) make copies of the statistics submitted to the Secretary available to the public; and

(C) in coordination with representatives of institutions of higher education, identify exemplary campus security policies, procedures, and practices and disseminate information concerning those policies, procedures, and practices that have proven effective in the reduction of campus crime.

(6)(A) In this subsection:

(i) The terms "dating violence," "domestic violence," and "stalking" have the meaning given such terms in section 40002(a) of the Violence Against Women Act of 1994 (42 U.S.C. 13925(a)).

The term "campus" means—

(I) any building or property owned or controlled by an institution of higher education within the same reasonably contiguous geographic area of the institution and used by the institution in direct support of, or in a manner related to, the institution's educational purposes, including residence halls; and property within the same reasonably contiguous geographic area of the institution that is owned by the institution but controlled by another person, is used by students, and supports institutional purposes (such as a food or other retail vendor).

(iii) The term "noncampus building or property" means—

(I) any building or property owned or controlled by a student organization recognized by the institution; and

(II) any building or property (other than a branch campus) owned or controlled by an institution of higher education that is used in direct support of, or in relation to, the institution's educational purposes, is used by students, and is not within the same reasonably contiguous geographic area of the institution.

(iv) The term "public property" means all public property that is within the same reasonably contiguous geographic area of the institution, such as a sidewalk, a street, other thorough- fare, or parking facility, and is adjacent to a facility owned or controlled by the institution if the facility is used by the institution in direct support of, or in a manner related to the institution's educational purposes.

(v) The term "sexual assault" means an offense classified as a forcible or nonforcible sex offense under the uniform crime reporting system of the Federal Bureau of Investigation.

(B) (B) In cases where branch campuses of an institution of higher education, schools within an institution of higher education, or administrative divisions within an institution are not within a reasonably contiguous geographic area, such entities shall be considered separate campuses for purposes of the reporting requirements of this section.

(7) The statistics described in clauses (i) and (ii) of paragraph (1)(F) shall be compiled in accordance with the definitions used in the uniform crime reporting system of the Department of Justice, Federal Bureau of Investigation, and the modifications in such definitions as implemented pursuant to the Hate Crime Statistics Act. For the offenses of domestic violence, dating violence, and stalking, such statistics shall be compiled in accordance with the definitions used in section 40002(a) of the Violence Against Women Act of 1994 (42 U.S.C. 13925(a)). Such statistics shall not identify victims of crimes or persons accused of crimes.

(8) (A) Each institution of higher education participating in any program under this title and title IV of the Economic Opportunity Act of 1964, other than a foreign institution of higher education, shall develop and distribute as part of the report described in paragraph (1) a statement of policy regarding—

(i) such institution's programs to prevent domestic violence, dating violence, sexual assault, and stalking; and

(ii) the procedures that such institution will follow once an incident of domestic violence, dating violence, sexual assault, or stalking has been reported, including a statement of the standard of evidence that will be used during any institutional conduct proceeding arising from such a report.

(B) The policy described in subparagraph (A) shall address the following areas:

(i) Education programs to promote the awareness of rape, acquaintance rape, domestic violence, dating violence, sexual assault, and stalking, which shall include—

(ii) primary prevention and awareness programs for all incoming students and new employees, which shall include—

(aa) a statement that the institution of higher education prohibits the offenses of domestic violence, dating violence, sexual assault, and stalking;

(bb) the definition of domestic violence, dating violence, sexual assault, and stalking in the applicable jurisdiction;

(cc) the definition of consent, in reference to sexual activity, in the applicable jurisdiction;

(dd) safe and positive options for bystander intervention that may be carried out by an individual to prevent harm or intervene when there is a risk of domestic violence, dating violence, sexual assault, or stalking against a person other than such individual; (ee) information on risk reduction to recognize warning signs of abusive behavior and how to avoid potential attacks; and

(ff) the information described in clauses (ii) through (vii); and

(I) ongoing prevention and awareness campaigns for students and faculty, including information described in items (aa) through (ff) of subclause (I).

(ii) Possible sanctions or protective measures that such institution may impose following a final determination of an institutional disciplinary procedure regarding rape, acquaintance rape, domestic violence, dating violence, sexual assault, or stalking.

(iii) Procedures victims should follow if a sex offense, domestic violence, dating violence, sexual assault, or stalking has occurred, including information in writing about—

(I) the importance of preserving evidence as may be necessary to the proof of criminal domestic violence, dating violence, sexual assault, or stalking, or in obtaining a protection order;

(II) to whom the alleged offense should be reported;

(III) options regarding law enforcement and campus authorities, including notification of the victim's option to— (aa) notify proper law enforcement authorities, including on-campus and local police;

(bb) be assisted by campus authorities in notifying law enforcement authorities if the victim so chooses; and

(cc) decline to notify such authorities; and

(IV) where applicable, the rights of victims and the institution's responsibilities regarding orders of protection, no contact orders, restraining orders, or similar lawful orders issued by a criminal, civil, or tribal court.

(iv) Procedures for institutional disciplinary action in cases of alleged domestic violence, dating violence, sexual assault, or stalking, which shall include a clear statement that—

(I) such proceedings shall—

(aa) provide a prompt, fair, and impartial investigation and resolution; and

(bb) be conducted by officials who receive annual training on the issues related to domestic violence, dating violence, sexual assault, and stalking and how to conduct an investigation and hearing process that protects the safety of victims and promotes accountability;

(cc) the accuser and the accused are entitled to the same opportunities to have others present during an institutional disciplinary proceeding, including the opportunity to be accompanied to any related meeting or proceeding by an advisor of their choice; and

(III) both the accuser and the accused shall be simultaneously informed, in writing, of—

(aa) the outcome of any institutional disciplinary proceeding that arises from an allegation of domestic violence, dating violence, sexual assault, or stalking;

(bb) the institution's procedures for the accused and the victim to appeal the results of the institutional disciplinary proceeding;

(cc) of any change to the results that occurs prior to the time that such results become final; and

(dd) when such results become final.

(v) Information about how the institution will protect the confidentiality of victims, including how publicly-available recordkeeping will be accomplished without the inclusion of identifying information about the victim, to the extent permissible by law.

(vi) Written notification of students and employees about existing counseling, health, mental health, victim advocacy, legal assistance, and other services available for victims both on-campus and in the community.

(vii) Written notification of victims about options for, and available assistance in, changing academic, living, transportation, and working situations, if so requested by the victim and if such accommodations are reasonably available, regardless of whether the victim chooses to report the crime to campus police or local law enforcement.

(C) A student or employee who reports to an institution of higher education that the student or employee has been a victim of domestic violence, dating violence, sexual assault, or stalking, whether the offense occurred on or off campus, shall be provided with a written explanation of the student or employee's rights and options, as described in clauses (ii) through (vii) of subparagraph (B).

(9) The Secretary, in consultation with the Attorney General of the United States, shall provide technical assistance in complying with the provisions of this section to an institution of higher education who requests such assistance.

(10) Nothing in this section shall be construed to require the reporting or disclosure of privileged information.

(11) The Secretary shall report to the appropriate committees of Congress each institution of higher education that the Secretary determines is not in compliance with the reporting requirements of this subsection.

(12) For purposes of reporting the statistics with respect to crimes described in paragraph (1)(F), an institution of higher education shall distinguish, by means of separate categories, any criminal offenses that occur—

(A) on campus;

(B)in or on a noncampus building or property;

(C)on public property; and

(D) in dormitories or other residential facilities for students on campus.

(13) Upon a determination pursuant to section 487(c)(3)(B) that an institution of higher education has substantially misrepresented the number, location, or nature of the crimes required to be reported under this subsection, the Secretary shall impose a civil penalty upon the institution in the same amount and pursuant to the same procedures as a civil penalty is imposed under section 487(c)(3)(B).

(14)(A) Nothing in this subsection may be construed to—

(i)create a cause of action against any institution of higher education or any employee of such an institution for any civil liability; or

(ii) establish any standard of care.

(B) Notwithstanding any other provision of law, evidence regarding compliance or noncompliance with this subsection shall not be admissible as evidence in any proceeding of any court, agency, board, or other entity, except with respect to an action to enforce this subsection.

(15) The Secretary shall annually report to the authorizing committees regarding compliance with this subsection by institutions of higher education,

including an up-to-date report on the Secretary's monitoring of such compliance.

(16)(A) The Secretary shall seek the advice and counsel of the Attorney General of the United States concerning the development, and dissemination to institutions of higher education, of best practices information about campus safety and emergencies.

(B) The Secretary shall seek the advice and counsel of the Attorney General of the United States and the Secretary of Health and Human Services concerning the development, and dissemination to institutions of higher education, of best practices information about preventing and responding to incidents of domestic violence, dating violence, sexual assault, and stalking, including elements of institutional policies that have proven successful based on evidence-based outcome measurements.

(17) No officer, employee, or agent of an institution participating in any program under this title shall retaliate, intimidate, threaten, coerce, or otherwise discriminate against any individual for exercising their rights or responsibilities under any provision of this subsection.

(18) This subsection may be cited as the "Jeanne Clery Disclosure of Campus Security Policy and Campus Crime Statistics Act."

(g) DATA REQUIRED.—

(1) IN GENERAL.—Each coeducational institution of higher education that participates in any program under this title, and has an intercollegiate athletic program, shall annually, for the immediately preceding academic year, prepare a report that contains the following information regarding intercollegiate athletics:

(A) The number of male and female full-time undergraduates that attended the institution.

(B) A listing of the varsity teams that competed in intercollegiate athletic competition and for each such team the following data:

(i) The total number of participants, by team, as of the day of the first scheduled contest for the team.

(ii) Total operating expenses attributable to such teams, except that an institution may also report such expenses on a per capita basis for each team and expenditures attributable to closely related teams such as track and field or swimming and diving, may be reported together, although such combinations shall be reported separately for men's and women's teams.

(iii) Whether the head coach is male or female and whether the head coach is assigned to that team on a full-time or part-time basis. Graduate assistants and volunteers who serve as head coaches shall be considered to be head coaches for the purposes of this clause.

(iv) The number of assistant coaches who are male and the number of assistant coaches who are female for each team and whether a particular coach is assigned to that team on a full-time or part-time basis. Graduate assistants and volunteers who serve as assistant coaches shall be considered to be assistant coaches for the purposes of this clause.

(C) The total amount of money spent on athletically related student aid, including the value of waivers of educational expenses, separately for men's and women's teams overall.

(D) The ratio of athletically related student aid awarded male athletes to athletically related student aid awarded female athletes.

(E) The total amount of expenditures on recruiting, separately for men's and women's teams overall.

(F) The total annual revenues generated across all men's teams and across all women's teams, except that an institution may also report such revenues by individual team.

(G) The average annual institutional salary of the head coaches of men's teams, across all offered sports, and the average annual institutional salary of the head coaches of women's teams, across all offered sports.

(H) The average annual institutional salary of the assistant coaches of men's teams, across all offered sports, and the average annual institutional salary of the assistant coaches of women's teams, across all offered sports.

(I)(i) The total revenues, and the revenues from football, men's basketball, women's basketball, all other men's sports combined and all other women's sports combined, derived by the institution from the institution's intercollegiate athletics activities.

(ii) For the purpose of clause (i), revenues from inter- collegiate athletics activities allocable to a sport shall include (without limitation) gate receipts, broadcast revenues, appearance guarantees and options, concessions, and advertising, but revenues such as student activities fees or alumni contributions not so allocable shall be included in the calculation of total revenues only.

(J)(i) The total expenses, and the expenses attributable to football, men's basketball, women's basketball, all other men's sports combined, and all other women's sports combined, made by the institution for the institution's intercollegiate athletics activities.

(ii) For the purpose of clause (i), expenses for intercollegiate athletics activities allocable to a sport shall include (without limitation) grants-in-aid, salaries, travel, equipment, and supplies, but expenses such as general and administrative overhead not so allocable shall be included in the calculation of total expenses only.

(2) SPECIAL RULE.—For the purposes of paragraph (1)(G), if a coach has responsibilities for more than one team and the institution does not allocate such coach's salary by team, the institution should divide the salary by the number of teams for which the coach has responsibility and allocate the salary among the teams on a basis consistent with the coach's responsibilities for the different teams.

(3) Disclosure of information to students and public.—

An institution of higher education described in paragraph (1) shall make available to students and potential students, upon request, and to the public, the information contained in the report described in paragraph (1), except that all students shall be informed of their right to request such information.

(4) SUBMISSION; REPORT; INFORMATION AVAILABILITY.—(A) On an annual basis, each institution of higher education described in paragraph (1) shall provide to the Secretary, within 15 days of the date that the institution makes available the report under paragraph (1), the information contained in the report.

(B) The Secretary shall ensure that the reports described in subparagraph (A) are made available to the public within a reasonable period of time.

(C) Not later than 180 days after the date of enactment of the Higher Education Amendments of 1998, the Secretary shall notify all secondary schools in all States regarding the availability of the information made available under paragraph (1), and how such information may be accessed.

(5) DEFINITION.—For the purposes of this subsection, the term "operating expenses" means expenditures on lodging and meals, transportation, officials, uniforms and equipment.

(h) TRANSFER OF CREDIT POLICIES.—

(1) DISCLOSURE.—Each institution of higher education participating in any program under this title shall publicly disclose, in a readable and comprehensible manner, the transfer of credit policies established by the institution which shall include a statement of the institution's current transfer of credit policies that includes, at a minimum—

(A)any established criteria the institution uses regarding the transfer of credit earned at another institution of higher education; and

(B) a list of institutions of higher education with which the institution has established an articulation agreement.

(2) RULE OF CONSTRUCTION.—Nothing in this subsection shall be construed to—

(A) authorize the Secretary or the National Advisory Committee on Institutional Quality and Integrity to require particular policies, procedures, or practices by institutions of higher education with respect to transfer of credit;

(B) authorize an officer or employee of the Department to exercise any direction, supervision, or control over the curriculum, program of instruction, administration, or personnel of any institution of higher education, or over any accrediting agency or association;

(C) limit the application of the General Education Provisions Act; or

(D) create any legally enforceable right on the part of a student to require an institution of higher education to accept a transfer of credit from another institution.

(i) DISCLOSURE OF FIRE SAFETY STANDARDS AND MEASURES.—

(1) Annual fire safety reports on student housing required.—Each eligible institution participating in any program under this title that maintains on-campus student housing facilities shall, on an annual basis, publish a fire safety report, which shall contain information with respect to the campus fire safety practices and standards of that institution, including—

(A) statistics concerning the following in each on-campus student housing facility during the most recent calendar years for which data are available:

(i)the number of fires and the cause of each fire;

(ii) the number of injuries related to a fire that result in treatment at a medical facility;

(iii) the number of deaths related to a fire; and

(iv) the value of property damage caused by a fire;

(B) a description of each on-campus student housing facility fire safety system, including the fire sprinkler system;

(C) the number of regular mandatory supervised fire drills;

(D) policies or rules on portable electrical appliances, smoking, and open flames (such as candles), procedures for evacuation, and policies regarding fire safety education and training programs provided to students, faculty, and staff; and

(E) plans for future improvements in fire safety, if determined necessary by such institution.

(2) REPORT TO THE SECRETARY.—Each institution described in paragraph (1) shall, on an annual basis, submit to the Secretary a copy of the statistics required to be made available under paragraph (1)(A).

(3) CURRENT INFORMATION TO CAMPUS COMMUNITY.—Each institution described in paragraph (1) shall—

(A) make, keep, and maintain a log, recording all fires in on-campus student housing facilities, including the nature, date, time, and general location of each fire; and

(B) make annual reports to the campus community on such fires.

(4) RESPONSIBILITIES OF THE SECRETARY.—The Secretary shall—

(A) make the statistics submitted under paragraph (1)(A) to the Secretary available to the public; and

(B) in coordination with nationally recognized fire organizations and representatives of institutions of higher education, representatives of associations of institutions of higher education, and other organizations that represent and house a significant number of students—

(i) identify exemplary fire safety policies, procedures, programs, and practices, including the installation, to the technical standards of the National Fire Protection Association, of fire detection, prevention, and protection technologies in student housing, dormitories, and other buildings;

(ii) disseminate the exemplary policies, procedures, programs and practices described in clause (i) to the Administrator of the United States Fire Administration;

(iii) make available to the public information concerning those policies, procedures, programs, and practices that have proven effective in the reduction of fires; and

(iv) develop a protocol for institutions to review the status of their fire safety systems.

(5) RULES OF CONSTRUCTION.—Nothing in this subsection shall be construed to—

(A) authorize the Secretary to require particular policies, procedures, programs, or practices by institutions of higher education with respect to fire safety, other than with respect to the collection, reporting, and dissemination of information required by this subsection;

(B) affect section 444 of the General Education Provisions Act (commonly known as the "Family Educational Rights and Privacy Act of 1974") or the regulations issued under section 264 of the Health Insurance Portability and Accountability Act of 1996 (42 U.S.C. 1320d–2 note);

(C) create a cause of action against any institution of higher education or any employee of such an institution for any civil liability; or

(D) establish any standard of care.

COMPLIANCE REPORT.—The Secretary shall annually report to the authorizing committees regarding compliance with this subsection by institutions of higher education, including an up-to-date report on the Secretary's monitoring of such compliance.

(7) EVIDENCE.—Notwithstanding any other provision of law, evidence regarding compliance or noncompliance with this subsection shall not be admissible as evidence in any proceeding of any court, agency, board, or other entity, except with respect to an action to enforce this subsection.

MISSING PERSON PROCEDURES.—

(1) OPTION AND PROCEDURES.—Each institution of higher education that provides on-campus housing and participates in any program under this title shall—

(A) establish a missing student notification policy for students who reside in on-campus housing that—

(i) informs each such student that such student has the option to identify an individual to be contacted by the institution not later than 24 hours after the time that the student is determined missing in accordance with official notification procedures established by the institution under subparagraph (B);

(ii) provides each such student a means to register confidential contact information in the event that the student is determined to be missing for a period of more than 24 hours;

(iii) advises each such student who is under 18 years of age, and not an emancipated individual, that the institution is required to notify a custodial parent or guardian not later 24 hours after the time that the student is determined to be missing in accordance with such procedures;

(iv) informs each such residing student that the institution will notify the appropriate law enforcement agency not later than 24 hours after the time that the student is determined missing in accordance with such procedures; and

(v) requires, if the campus security or law enforcement personnel has been notified and makes a determination that a student who is the subject of a missing person report has been missing for more than 24 hours and has not returned to the campus, the institution to initiate the emergency contact procedures in accordance with the student's designation; and

(B) establish official notification procedures for a missing student who resides in on-campus housing that—

(i) includes procedures for official notification of appropriate individuals at the institution that such student has been missing for more than 24 hours;

(ii) requires any official missing person report relating to such student be referred immediately to the institution's police or campus security department; and

(iii) if, on investigation of the official report, such department determines that the missing student has been missing for more than 24 hours, requires—

(I) such department to contact the individual identified by such student under subparagraph (A)(i);

(II) if such student is under 18 years of age, and not an emancipated individual, the institution to immediately contact the custodial parent or legal guardian of such student; and

(III) if subclauses (I) or (II) do not apply to a student determined to be a missing person, inform the appropriate law enforcement agency.

(2) RULE OF CONSTRUCTION.—Nothing in this subsection shall be construed—

(A) to provide a private right of action to any person to enforce any provision of this subsection; or

(B) to create a cause of action against any institution of higher education or any employee of the institution for any civil liability.

(k) NOTICE TO STUDENTS CONCERNING PENALTIES FOR DRUG VIOLATIONS.—

(1) NOTICE UPON ENROLLMENT.—Each institution of higher education shall provide to each student, upon enrollment, a separate, clear, and conspicuous written notice that advises the student of the penalties under section 484(r).

(2) NOTICE AFTER LOSS OF ELIGIBILITY.—An institution of higher education shall provide in a timely manner to each student who has lost eligibility for any grant, loan, or work-study assistance under this title as a result of the penalties listed under section 484(r)(1) a separate, clear, and conspicuous written notice that notifies the student of the loss of eligibility and advises the student of the ways in which the student can regain eligibility under section 484(r)(2).

(l) ENTRANCE COUNSELING FOR BORROWERS.—

(1) Disclosure required prior to disbursement.—

(A) IN GENERAL.—Each eligible institution shall, at or prior to the time of a disbursement to a first-time borrower of a loan made, insured, or guaranteed under part B (other than a loan made pursuant to section 428C or a loan made on behalf of a student pursuant to section 428B) or made under part D (other than a Federal Direct Consolidation Loan or a Federal Direct PLUS loan made on behalf of a student), ensure that the borrower receives comprehensive information on the terms and conditions of the loan and of the responsibilities the borrower has with respect to such loan in accordance with paragraph (2). Such information—

(i) shall be provided in a simple and understandable manner; and

(ii) may be provided—

(I) during an entrance counseling session conduction in person;

(II) on a separate written form provided to the borrower that the borrower signs and returns to the institution; or

(III) online, with the borrower acknowledging receipt of the information.

(B) USE OF INTERACTIVE PROGRAMS.—The Secretary shall encourage institutions to carry out the requirements of subparagraph (A) through the use of interactive programs that test the borrower's understanding of the terms and conditions of the borrower's loans under part B or D, using simple and understandable language and clear formatting.

(2) INFORMATION TO BE PROVIDED.—The information to be provided to the borrower under paragraph (1)(A) shall include the following:

(A) To the extent practicable, the effect of accepting the loan to be disbursed on the eligibility of the borrower for other forms of student financial assistance.

(B) An explanation of the use of the master promissory note.

(C) Information on how interest accrues and is capitalized during periods when the interest is not paid by either the borrower or the Secretary.

(D) In the case of a loan made under section 428B or 428H, a Federal Direct PLUS Loan, or a Federal Direct Unsubsidized Stafford Loan, the option of the borrower to pay the interest while the borrower is in school.

(E) The definition of half-time enrollment at the institution, during regular terms and summer school, if applicable, and the consequences of not maintaining half-time enrollment.

(F) An explanation of the importance of contacting the appropriate offices at the institution of higher education if the borrower withdraws prior to completing the borrower's program of study so that the institution can provide exit counseling, including information regarding the borrower's repayment options and loan consolidation.

(G) Sample monthly repayment amounts based on—

(i) a range of levels of indebtedness of—

(I) borrowers of loans under section 428 or 428H; and

(II) as appropriate, graduate borrowers of loans under section 428, 428B, or 428H; or

(ii) the average cumulative indebtedness of other borrowers in the same program as the borrower at the same institution.

(H) The obligation of the borrower to repay the full amount of the loan, regardless of whether the borrower completes or does not complete the program in which the borrower is enrolled within the regular time for program completion.

(I) The likely consequences of default on the loan, including adverse credit reports, delinquent debt collection procedures under Federal law, and litigation.

(J) Information on the National Student Loan Data System and how the borrower can access the borrower's records.

(K) The name of and contact information for the individual the borrower may contact if the borrower has any questions about the borrower's rights and responsibilities or the terms and conditions of the loan.

(m) DISCLOSURES OF REIMBURSEMENTS FOR SERVICE ON ADVISORY Boards.—

(1) DISCLOSURE.—Each institution of higher education participating in any program under this title shall report, on an annual basis, to the Secretary, any reasonable expenses paid or provided under section 140(d) of the Truth in Lending Act to any employee who is employed in the financial aid office of the institution, or who otherwise has responsibilities with respect to education loans or other financial aid of the institution. Such reports shall include—

(A) the amount for each specific instance of reasonable expenses paid or provided;

(B) the name of the financial aid official, other employee, or agent to whom the expenses were paid or provided;

(C) the dates of the activity for which the expenses were paid or provided; and

(D) a brief description of the activity for which the expenses were paid or provided.

(2) REPORT TO CONGRESS.—The Secretary shall summarize the information received from institutions of higher education under paragraph (1) in a report and transmit such report annually to the authorizing committees.

(n) PREGNANT STUDENTS' RIGHTS, ACCOMMODATIONS, AND RESOURCES.—

(1) IN GENERAL.—Each institution of higher education participating in any program under this title shall carry out the information dissemination activities described in paragraph (3) for prospective and enrolled students (including those attending or planning to attend less than full time) regarding

the information described in paragraph (2) on the rights to, and resources (including protections and accommodations) for, pregnant students to carry a baby to term and students who may become pregnant while enrolled at such institution of higher education to carry a baby to term.

(2) INFORMATION CONTENT.—The information described in this paragraph is the following:

(A) A list of resources on campus and in the community that exist to help a pregnant student in carrying the baby to term and caring for the baby after birth.

(B) Information about the accommodations available to help a pregnant student carry the baby to term and parent the baby after birth.

(C) Information on how to file a complaint with—

(i) the Department of Education, if a student believes there was a violation by the institution of title IX of the Education Amendments of 1972 (20 U.S.C. 1681 et seq.) on account of such student's determination to carry a baby to term; and

(ii) the institution, if a student believes the student has been discriminated against in violation of such title IX on account of the student's determination to carry a baby to term.

(3) INFORMATION DISSEMINATION ACTIVITIES.—The information dissemination activities described in this paragraph shall include—

(A) an email to each enrolled student at the start of each period of study during an academic year; and the provision of information—

(i) in student handbooks, if any;

(ii) at each orientation for enrolled students;

(iii) at student health or counseling centers, if any; and

(iv) on the publicly available website of the institution of higher education.

(4) RULE OF CONSTRUCTION.—Nothing in this subsection shall be construed to authorize the Secretary to require the dissemination of additional information, or establish additional rights, beyond the information and rights included in this subsection.

* * * * * * *

Minority Views

H.R. 6914, the Pregnant Students' Rights Act, introduced by Rep. Ashley Hinson (R–IA), requires institutions of higher education, as a condition of their receipt of funds under Title IV of the Higher Education Act,[20] to inform potential and current students of the rights and resources available for pregnant students to carry a baby to term and students who may become pregnant. On its face, this bill may appear to ensure students are well-informed about available resources and the ways students can continue to access their education while pregnant, but in fact, it is an attempt to dissuade students from considering or utilizing abortion services and make it more difficult for students to receive full and accurate information on their rights. This is why dozens of health and reproductive rights organizations have asserted that the bill "falls far short of the protections that are actually necessary for pregnant and parenting students and their children" and "is a thinly veiled anti-abortion [bill] which would not address the key barriers to pregnant students' educational attainment, and instead would further shame and stigmatize people for their pregnancy outcomes."[21] The Pregnant Students' Rights Act explicitly requires that the information shared with potential and current students be related to carrying a baby to term and caring for a baby after birth. The bill conspicuously omits any requirement for institutions of higher education to distribute medically accurate and comprehensive information regarding pregnancy, including information on abortion services. Nor does the bill require these schools to provide information on access to comprehensive sexual health and reproductive health services, including contraception, which could help students avoid unplanned pregnancies. Importantly, the bill fails to require schools to provide information on rights and resources for students who terminate a pregnancy or students who face a pregnancy loss. Troublingly, the bill does not provide any additional resources or grant additional rights to pregnant and parenting students, leaving those the bill purports to help with the same inadequate resources, such as unaffordable child care, as without the bill.

Section 2 of the bill includes a number of anti-abortion findings, which allege without supporting data, in part, that "female students enrolled at institutions of higher education and experiencing an unplanned pregnancy

---

[20] Higher Education Act of 1965, Pub. L. No. 89–329, as amended.

[21] Letter to the Honorable Virginia Foxx and the Honorable Robert ''Bobby'' Scott from the Coalition for Pregnant and Parenting Students Advocacy, et. al (Jan. 10, 2024), *on file with author*.

may face pressure that their only option is to receive an abortion or risk academic failure."[22] Unfortunately, the Committee adopted an amendment offered by Rep. Bob Good (R–VA) adding a number of unsubstantiated claims regarding the purported harms of abortion to the findings section. During the Committee's consideration of the Good amendment, an inquiry was made by Rep. Suzanne Bonamici (D–OR) to provide sources for the claims in the findings. Rep. Good was unable to provide the source for the information.

It is worth noting that longstanding regulations implementing Title IX of the Education Amendments of 1972[23] (Title IX), which prohibits discrimination on the basis of sex in education programs or activities that receive federal funding, forbid discriminating against students on the basis of the student's pregnancy, childbirth, false pregnancy, termination of pregnancy, or recovery therefrom.[24] These requirements ensure that students are not denied or otherwise limited access to educational programs or activities based on their pregnancy or related medical conditions. The U.S. Department of Education (Department) recognizes the role that Title IX plays in protecting pregnant students. In fact, in October 2022, the Department issued a resource to students and schools to reinforce protections for pregnancy and related medical conditions, including abortion, under Title IX in light of the Supreme Court's ruling in Dobbs v. Jackson Women's Health Organization.[25] Specifically, the Department indicated that relevant regulations "provide . . . [that] schools must not discriminate against any student, or exclude any student from their education program or activity, including any class or extracurricular activity, based on a student's pregnancy, childbirth, false pregnancy, termination of pregnancy, or recovery therefrom."[26] Therefore,

---

[22] Pregnant Students' Rights Act, H.R. 6915, 118th Cong. § 2 (2024).

[23] Education Amendments of 1972, Pub. L. No. 92–318, § § 901–07, 86 Stat. 235, 373–74 (1972).

[24] 34 C.F.R. § § 106.21, 106.40, 106.51, 106.57. The verbatim language first appeared in the 1975 regulations implementing Title IX promulgated in 45 C.F.R. § § 86.21, 40, 51, 57 for the U.S. Department of Health, Education, and Welfare. (Nondiscrimination on the Basis of Sex in Education Programs and Activities Receiving or Benefiting from Federal Financial Assistance, 40 Fed. Reg. 24128 (June 4, 1975) (codified at 45 C.F.R. pt. 86).) These regulations were subject to a statutory ''laying before'' provision which afforded Congress the opportunity to review and possibly reject the regulations within a 45 day period if found to be inconsistent with Title IX. Ultimately, Congress did not disapprove of the regulations. In *Grove City College v. Bell*, the U.S. Supreme Court found that Congress' failure to act ''strongly implies'' that the regulations reflect congressional intent. (*Grove City Coll. v. Bell*, 465 U.S. 555, 568 (1984).)

[25] Dobbs v. Jackson Women's Health Organization, 597 U.S. 215 (2022).

[26] U.S. Department of Education Office of Civil Rights, Discrimination Based on Pregnancy and Related Conditions A Resource for Students and Schools, ED OCR (Oct. 4, 2022), https://www2.ed.gov/about/offices/list/ocr/docs/ocr-pregnancy-resource. pdf.

current law protects students from discriminatory actions regarding pregnancy in educational settings. Further, in 2022 the Department issued a proposed rule to strengthen Title IX protections, including a number of substantive steps to support students regarding a full range of pregnancy related conditions.[27] For example, the proposed rule strengthens training requirements for employees, including the Title IX Coordinator at the respective institutions of higher education, on their obligations to pregnant and parenting students.[28] To support student parents who are nursing, the proposed rule adds "lactation" as a related condition alongside childbirth and other pregnancy related conditions that should be protected under Title IX to ensure that parenting students can receive accommodations, including access to lactation space.[29] In addition, the proposed rule requires employees who become aware of a student's pregnancy or related condition to connect that student with the school's Title IX Coordinator,[30] and subsequently, requires those Title IX Coordinators to notify those students of their rights under Title IX.[31] Importantly, the proposed rule offers substantive and meaningful updates to strengthen Title IX's protections of students who are pregnant or experiencing pregnancy related conditions.

Committee Democrats remain committed to ensuring that all students—including those who choose to become parents—are set up for educational success. Students undeniably face a host of challenges during their academic pursuits. Research, including reports from the Government Accountability Office (GAO), have assessed the challenges of students' meeting basic needs and costs of living[32] as well as high child care costs for parenting students.[33] Low-income parenting students often face barriers to finding affordable child care services.[34] In short, much more needs to be done to support the financial

---

[27] Nondiscrimination on the Basis of Sex in Education Programs or Activities Receiving Federal Financial Assistance, 87 Fed. Reg. 41390 (proposed July 12, 2022) (to be codified at 34 C.F.R. pt. 106), ttps://federalregister.gov/d/2022-13734.

[28] *Id.* at 41570 (proposed 34 C.F.R. § 106.8(d)).

[29] *Id.* at 41568 (proposed 34 C.F.R. § 106.2).

[30] *Id.* at 41571 (proposed 34 C.F.R. § 106.40(b)(2).

[31] *Id.* at 41571–72 (proposed 34 C.F.R. § 106.40(b)(3)(i)).

[32] *Better Information Could Help Eligible College Students Access Federal Food Assistance Benefits,* U.S. Government Accountability Office (Jan. 9, 2019), https://www.gao.gov/products/ gao-19-95.

[33] *Information Could Help Student Parents Access Additional Federal Student Aid,* U.S. Government Accountability Office (Sept. 12, 2019), https://www.gao.gov/products/gao-19-522.

[34] Brittani Williams, Jinann Bitar, Portia Polk, Andre Nguyen, Gabriel Montague, Carrie Gillispie, Antoinette Waller, Azeb Tadesse, and Kayla C. Elliott, *For Student Parents, The Big- gest Hurdles to A Higher Education are Costs and Finding Child Care,* The Education

security of our nation's students. Committee Democrats have introduced numerous pieces of legislation that would better support parents—including students who are parents—such as through the expansion of affordable child care[35] and raising the federal minimum wage to provide family-sustaining pay.[36]

Preserving access to quality and comprehensive reproductive health care is also critical for the overall wellbeing and academic success of all students, including those who are pregnant or parenting. For over a decade, the Affordable Care Act (ACA)[37] has increased the number of affordable health coverage options available to students and their families, including those who rely on access to contraception, prenatal care, and other essential health care services. Unfortunately, anti-choice efforts, such as those underpinning this bill, only make it harder for students to succeed, and many students are experiencing new and added stress when navigating their health and access to health care. In the wake of Dobbs, many states have prohibited health care providers from offering certain reproductive health care services.[38] New state restrictions have limited access to contraception and other preventive services as well as the availability of providers.[39] Some students may be disproportionately affected by geographical barriers unique to their institutions that only reinforce structural inequities. For example, approximately 80 percent of Historically Black Colleges and Universities (HBCUs) are located in states that have passed restrictions or bans on abortion care, pushing services further out of reach for hundreds of thousands of students.[40]

Trust (Aug. 17, 2022), https://edtrust.org/resource/for-student-parents-the-biggest-hurdles-to-a-higher-education-are-costs-and-finding-child-care/.

[35] Child Care for Working Families Act, H.R. 2976, 118th Cong. (2023).

[36] Raise the Wage Act of 2023, H.R. 4889, 118th Cong. (2023).

[37] 42 U.S.C. 300gg–14.

[38] Kimya Forouzan & Isabel Guarnieri, State Policy Trends 2023: In the First Full Year Since Roe Fell, a Tumultuous Year for Abortion and Other Reproductive Health Care, The Guttmacher Institute (Dec. 2023), https://www.guttmacher.org/2023/ 12/state-policy-trends-2023-first-full-year-roe-fell-tumultuous-year-abortion-and-other.

[39] *See*, Max G. Levy, *At Some Colleges, the Fall of Roe Will Weaken Student Health Care,* WIRED (Aug. 23, 2022), https://www.wired.com/story/at-some-colleges-the-fall-of-roe-will-weaken-student-health-care/; Oriana Gonza´lez, *Post-Dobbs birth control fight heads to college campuses,* AXIOS (Oct. 2, 2022), https://www.axios.com/2022/09/30/dobbs-roe-abortion-university-birth- control; Julie Rovner, *Abortion bans drive off doctors and close clinics, putting other health care at risk,* NPR (May 23, 2023), https://www.npr.org/sections/health-shots/2023/05/23/1177542605/abortion-bans-drive-off-doctors-and-put-other-health-care-at-risk.

[40] *See*, Lauren Lumpkin, *HBCU students are being disproportionately affected by Roe's reversal,* THE WASHINGTON POST (Jul. 20, 2022), https://www.washing tonpost.com/

During the markup of H.R. 6914, Committee Democrats re-affirmed their commitment to ensuring that students have the tools and resources they need to succeed. Democratic Members of the Committee offered amendments to ensure that students receive more comprehensive and well-rounded information about their rights and available resources. Specifically, Rep. Bonamici offered an amendment to add a rule of construction that would ensure that nothing in the bill prevents institutions of higher education from providing medically accurate and comprehensive information about abortion services. Rep. Kathy Manning (D–NC) offered an amendment to add a rule of construction that would clarify that nothing in the bill prevents schools from providing students information on access to comprehensive sexual health and reproductive health services, including contraception. To better ensure that pregnant students would receive helpful information on services to support them, Rep. Pramila Jayapal (D–WA) offered an amendment to add a requirement to provide information on access to federal programs that support the health and wellbeing of pregnant women and children, including Medicaid, the Supplemental Nutrition Assistance Program (SNAP), Title X of the Public Health Service Act,[41] and the Special Supplemental Nutrition Program for Women, Infants, and Children (WIC). Rep. Haley Stevens (D–MI) offered an amendment to add a rule of construction that would clarify that nothing in the bill prevents schools from disseminating information on resources (including available rights, protections, and accommodations afforded to students under Title IX) regarding pregnancy and related medical conditions, including miscarriage. Committee Republicans rejected all of these Democratic amendments. Finally, Rep. Jahana Hayes (D–CT) offered an amendment to expand the Child Tax Credit (CTC); the amendment was withdrawn.

House Republicans have been relentless in their attempts to take away reproductive freedom. They have attempted to "defund" Planned Parenthood,[42] which would prevent people from accessing critical preventive services such as breast and cervical cancer screenings, and eliminate funding

---

education/2022/07/ 20/abortion-access-hbcus-roevwade/; Caroline Kitchener et al., *States where abortion is legal, banned or under threat,* THE WASHINGTON POST, https://www.washingtonpost.com/politics/2022/06/24/abortion-state-laws-criminalization-roe/ (last visited Jan. 5, 2024). Since July 20, 2022, North Carolina and Florida have enacted abortion bans and Ohio has reversed its law; the number of HBCUs impacted increased from 72 to at least 80.

[41] 42 U.S.C. 300 *et seq.*

[42] Making appropriations for the Departments of Labor, Health and Human Services, and Education, and related agencies for the fiscal year ending September 30, 2024, and for other purposes, H.R. 5894, 118th Cong. § 240 (2023).

for the Teen Pregnancy Prevention Program (TPPP), which provides honest and accurate sex edu cation programs to prevent unintended pregnancies.[43] Not only have Republicans directly targeted reproductive rights, they have relentlessly targeted the programs and services that actually support women, children, and families. For example, the Republicans' Fiscal Year 2024 Agriculture appropriations bill proposed drastic cuts to WIC,[44] despite the increased need facing parents and children. Republican opposition to expansions of the CTC included in the American Rescue Plan Act of 2021,[45] which increased the value of the credit and crucially ensured that the full value of the credit was available to all lower- and middle-income families, allowed those temporary provisions to expire.[46] The CTC alone was estimated to have kept 2.1 million children out of poverty in 2021.[47] If the expanded CTC were reinstated in 2024, nearly 60 million children would benefit.[48] In addition, the House Republicans' Labor, Health and Human Services, Education, and Related Agencies appropriations bill for Fiscal Year 2024 cuts billions in programs that support education, job opportunities, and maternal health.[49]

H.R. 6914 is not an earnest attempt to support students. As we continue to fight for abortion rights and reproductive autonomy, we must ensure that students are fully informed of all options regarding their reproductive health and wellness. At the same time, it is important to recognize that Title IX

---

[43] See House Committee on Appropriations—Chairwoman Kay Granger, Explanatory Materials for the Departments of Labor, Health and Human Services, and Education, and Related Agencies Appropriations Bill, 2024—H.R. 5894 (2023), https://appropriations.house.gov/sites/republicans.appropriations.house.gov/files/FY24-LHHS-Explanatory-Materials.pdf.

[44] Katie Bergh & Lauren Hall, Looming WIC Funding Shortfall Would Jeopardize Access to WIC's Proven Benefits and Disproportionately Harm Black and Hispanic Families, CTR. ON BUDGET AND POL'Y PRIORITIES (Oct. 26, 2023), https://www.cbpp.org/blog/looming-wic-funding-shortfall-would-jeopardize-access-to-wics-proven-benefits-and.

[45] American Rescue Plan Act of 2021, Pub. L. No. 117–2.

[46] Joe Hughes and Emma Sifre, Expanding the Child Tax Credit Would Advance Racial Eq- uity in the Tax Code, INST. ON TAX'N AND ECON. POL'Y (Aug. 29, 2023), https://itep.org/expanding-the-child-tax-credit-would-advance-racial-equity-in-the-tax-code/.

[47] Joe Hughes, Census Data Shows Need to Make 2021 Child Tax Credit Expansion Perma- nent, INST. ON TAX'N AND ECON. POL'Y (Sept. 14. 2022), https://itep.org/census-data-shows-need-to-make-2021-child-tax-credit-expansion-permanent/.

[48] Joe Hughes and Emma Sifre, Expanding the Child Tax Credit Would Advance Racial Equity in the Tax Code, INST. ON TAX'N AND ECON. POL'Y (Aug. 29, 2023), https://itep.org/expanding-the-child-tax-credit-would-advance-racial-equity-in-the-tax-code/.

[49] House Committee on Appropriations—Ranking Member Rosa DeLauro, Fact Sheet: Labor, Health and Human Services, Education, and Related Agencies (2023), https://democrats-appropriations.house.gov/sites/democrats.appropriations.house.gov/files/FY24%20LHHS%20Summary.pdf.

protects pregnant students' ability to pursue an education. For these reasons, we urge the House of Representatives to oppose H.R. 6914.

Robert C. "Bobby" Scott,
Ranking Member. Rau´ l M. Grijalva, Joe Courtney,
Gregorio Kilili Camacho Sablan,
Frederica S. Wilson, Suzanne Bonamici, Mark Takano,
Alma S. Adams, Mark DeSaulnier, Donald Norcross,
Pramila Jayapal, Susan Wild, Lucy McBath,
Haley M. Stevens, Teresa Leger Fernandez, Kathy E. Manning,
Frank J. Mrvan,
Jamaal Bowman,
Members of Congress.

Chapter 8

Pregnancy and Labor: An Overview of Federal Laws Protecting Pregnant Workers*

April J. Anderson

Summary

Several different federal laws protect workers from discrimination based on pregnancy. The oldest of these, the Pregnancy Discrimination Act (PDA), generally protects job applicants and employees from adverse action—for example, firing, demotion, refusal to hire, or forced leave—because of pregnancy or related conditions. The PDA also addresses harassment based on pregnancy and bans retaliation against workers for making complaints about pregnancy discrimination. Pregnancy-related conditions can include fertility treatments, medical complications, delivery, postpartum conditions, and lactation. The PDA was enacted as an amendment to Title VII of the Civil Rights Act of 1964, which protects against sex discrimination (as well as certain other forms of discrimination) in employment.

As construed by the Supreme Court, the PDA does not generally require employers to make changes in working conditions to accommodate pregnant workers unless employers provide accommodations to other similarly situated nonpregnant workers. So, while employers cannot fire workers for being pregnant, this statute (depending on the facts) may not require them to make workplace changes (e.g., scheduling flexibility, an extra bathroom break) simply because employees' demands are pregnancy-related.

* This is an edited, reformatted and augmented version of Congressional Research Service Publication No. R46821, dated July 3, 2023.

In: Navigating Pregnancy Challenges
Editor: Javier Giles
ISBN: 979-8-89530-857-8

The Pregnant Workers Fairness Act (PWFA), passed in 2022 and effective June 27, 2023, mandates additional protections for pregnant workers. Modeled on the Americans with Disabilities Act (ADA), it requires employers to modify workplace conditions where needed to accommodate pregnancy-related conditions as long as an accommodation is reasonable and does not present an undue hardship to the employer. The PWFA requires a reasonable accommodation, after a case-specific assessment, even if a pregnancy-related condition does not amount to a disability, and even if the accommodation includes reassignment of an essential job function. Relief from an essential job function is only required, however, if it is temporary. In addition, under the PWFA, an employer may not require an employee to take leave if a reasonable accommodation would allow her to keep working.

Some pregnant people face pregnancy-related impairments serious enough to satisfy the ADA's definition of a "disability" and may, along with any PDA or PWFA claims, bring ADA claims for accommodations. Separately, many workers can invoke the Family and Medical Leave Act (FMLA) for unpaid leave for pregnancy-related medical needs. After childbirth, provisions of the Fair Labor Standards Act (FLSA) entitle most nursing mothers to appropriate breaks and accommodations for expressing breast milk.

Preceding the passage of the PWFA, many advocates and legislators proposed expanding legal protections for pregnancy. Proposals included new pregnancy accommodation requirements (modeled on disability law), antidiscrimination measures (expanding current statutes), and leave entitlements (in line with many analogous mandates for reemployment rights or leave entitlements to protect workers engaged in endeavors such as military service). The PWFA focused on this first approach: accommodations. In addition, many states have strengthened rights for pregnant workers in recent years, and the PWFA does not preempt those laws when they offer greater protection.

Introduction

Federal laws have protected pregnant workers for decades. These laws generally bar employers from taking adverse action against a worker because of pregnancy. Historically, these laws did not typically require employers to make workplace changes to accommodate pregnancy, unless such accommodations were provided to similarly situated, nonpregnant workers, or unless pregnancy impairments amounted to a disability. The Pregnant Workers Fairness Act (PWFA), passed in 2022 and effective June 27, 2023, requires accommodations for most pregnant workers.

The Equal Employment Opportunity Commission (EEOC), the federal entity mainly charged with monitoring compliance and enforcing antidiscrimination laws in employment, reports that it receives thousands of pregnancy discrimination complaints each year.[1] The majority of charges of pregnancy discrimination allege that individuals faced termination based on pregnancy.[2] Other charges include claims that pregnant workers endured harsher discipline, suspensions pending receipt of medical releases, suggestions that they undergo an abortion, and involuntary leave.[3]

This report provides an overview of laws protecting pregnant workers, including their substantive provisions, legislative history, practical considerations, judicial interpretation, and limitations. In addition, this report summarizes proposed pregnancy protections and describes other employment laws that may serve as models for potential legislation.

Federal Law Prior to the Pregnancy Discrimination Act

Before the enactment of the Pregnancy Discrimination Act (PDA), federal law did not expressly address the discriminatory treatment of pregnant workers. The primary federal statute addressing discrimination in the workplace, Title VII of the Civil Rights Act of 1964, makes it unlawful to discriminate "against any individual with respect to his compensation, terms, conditions, or privileges of employment, because of such individual's . . . sex."[4] Prohibited actions include discharge, discrimination in pay, denial of promotion,

---

[1] U.S. EQUAL EMP. OPPORTUNITY COMM'N, PREGNANCY DISCRIMINATION CHARGES FY 2010–FY 2021 [hereinafter EEOC], https://www.eeoc.gov/data/pregnancy-discrimination-charges-FY-2010-FY-2021 (last visited June 7, 2023).

[2] U.S. EQUAL EMP. OPPORTUNITY COMM'N, ENFORCEMENT GUIDANCE ON PREGNANCY DISCRIMINATION AND RELATED ISSUES, No. 915.003 (June 25, 2015) [hereinafter EEOC Enforcement Guidance], https://www.eeoc.gov/laws/guidance/enforcement-guidance-pregnancy-discrimination-and-related-issues (last visited June 7, 2023).

[3] *Id.*; Joan Williams, *Written Testimony of Joan Williams Professor of Law UC Hastings Foundation Chair Director, Center for Worklife Law – Unlawful Discrimination Against Pregnant Workers and Workers with Caregiving Responsibilities*, U.S. EQUAL EMP. OPPORTUNITY COMM'N (February 15, 2012), http://www.eeoc.gov/eeoc/meetings/2-15-12/williams.cfm.

[4] 42 U.S.C. § 2000e-2(a)(1) ("It shall be an unlawful employment practice for an employer to fail or refuse to hire or to discharge any individual, or otherwise to discriminate against any individual with respect to his compensation, terms, conditions, or privileges of employment, because of such individual's race, color, religion, sex, or national origin."); EEOC ENFORCEMENT GUIDANCE, *supra* note 2.

demotion, harsher discipline, suspensions, and forced leave.[5] Along with adverse actions, Title VII bars harassment because of sex—that is, harsh treatment severe or pervasive enough to alter the employee's terms and conditions of employment.[6] Title VII also protects workers from retaliation when they oppose discrimination, file a discrimination complaint, or participate in the complaint.[7] If they prevail on a claim of discrimination or retaliation, employees may seek equitable relief and damages, including back pay and punitive damages.[8]

Because (in its original form) Title VII did not mention pregnancy, courts were left to determine how the prohibition on sex discrimination applied to pregnant workers. In 1976, the Supreme Court took up the issue in General Electric Co. v. Gilbert. In that case, General Electric offered a benefits plan to compensate employees unable to work because of illness or injury.[9] The plan excluded pregnancy and related conditions, but not other medical conditions, from coverage.[10] After a class of women employees presented claims for pregnancy-related medical conditions and challenged the plan as discriminatory, the Court held that the pregnancy exclusion did not violate Title VII because it did not treat men and women differently.[11] The benefits plan did not divide employees into groups of men and groups of women for separate treatment, as the Court saw it; instead, the plan separated employees into groups of pregnant and nonpregnant people.[12] The Court said that "[n]ormal pregnancy is an objectively identifiable physical condition with unique characteristics," and Title VII did not bar employers from excluding

---

[5] EEOC ENFORCEMENT GUIDANCE, *supra* note 2.

[6] Mendoza v. Borden, Inc., 195 F.3d 1238, 1245 (11th Cir. 1999); *see also* Harris v. Forklift Sys., Inc., 510 U.S. 17, 21(1993) (noting discrimination "includes requiring people to work in a discriminatorily hostile or abusive environment"); U.S. EQUAL EMP. OPPORTUNITY COMM'N, HARASSMENT, https://www.eeoc.gov/harassment (last visited June 7, 2023).

[7] 42 U.S.C. § 2000e-3(a); EEOC ENFORCEMENT GUIDANCE, *supra* note 2; U.S. EQUAL EMP. OPPORTUNITY COMM'N, QUESTIONS AND ANSWERS: ENFORCEMENT GUIDANCE ON RETALIATION AND RELATED ISSUES, https://www.eeoc.gov/laws/guidance/questions-and-answers-enforcement-guidance-retaliation-and-related-issues (last visited June 7, 2023).

[8] 42 U.S.C. § 1981; Kolstad v. Am. Dental Ass'n, 527 U.S. 526, 529 (1999); U.S. EQUAL EMP. OPPORTUNITY COMM'N, REMEDIES FOR EMPLOYMENT DISCRIMINATION, https://www.eeoc.gov/remedies-employment-discrimination (last visited June 7, 2023).

[9] Gen. Elec. Co. v. Gilbert, 429 U.S. 125, 127 (1976), *superseded by statute*, Pregnancy Discrimination Act of 1978, Pub. L. No. 95–555, 92 Stat. 2076 (1978), *as recognized in* Cal. Fed. Sav. & Loan Ass'n v. Guerra, 479 U.S. 272, 284–85 (1987).

[10] *Id.* at 127.

[11] *Id.* at 139.

[12] *Id.* at 135.

pregnancy from benefits coverage "on any reasonable basis."[13] The outcome might be different if the employer intended to target women for mistreatment, the Court acknowledged, but it concluded that General Electric's decision to exclude pregnancy was not pretext for sex discrimination.[14]

The Pregnancy Discrimination Act

In response to Gilbert, Congress passed the Pregnancy Discrimination Act as an amendment to Title VII. The PDA did not alter Title VII's provisions on remedies or enforcement. Instead, the PDA added two phrases to Title VII's definitions section clarifying that pregnancy discrimination is a form of sex discrimination.[15] The first phrase of the PDA adds pregnancy to the list of categories protected from discrimination, declaring that "[t]he terms 'because of sex' or 'on the basis of sex' include, but are not limited to, because of or on the basis of pregnancy, childbirth, or related medical conditions."[16] In light of this language, Title VII now expressly protects covered employees and job applicants from discrimination, including demotion, firing, the denial of employment, or harassment, based on pregnancy.[17]

In a second phrase, the PDA requires that "women affected by pregnancy, childbirth, or related medical conditions shall be treated the same for all employment-related purposes, including receipt of benefits under fringe benefit programs, as other persons not so affected but similar in their ability or inability to work."[18] Legislative history suggests that Congress intended the amendment to clarify that "distinctions based on pregnancy are per se violations of Title VII."[19]

---

[13] *Id.* at 134.

[14] *Id.* at 134–35.

[15] Cal. Fed. Sav. & Loan Ass'n v. Guerra, 479 U.S. 272, 284–85 (1987) (noting "the PDA reflects Congress' disapproval of the reasoning in *Gilbert*"); *see also* Newport News Shipbuilding & Dry Dock Co. v. EEOC, 462 U.S. 669, 681 (1983) (observing that "[p]roponents of the legislation stressed throughout the debates that Congress had always intended to protect *all* individuals from sex discrimination in employment—including but not limited to pregnant women workers").

[16] 42 U.S.C. § 2000e(k).

[17] *Id.* §§ 2000e(k), 2000e-2; EEOC ENFORCEMENT GUIDANCE, *supra* note 2.

[18] 42 U.S.C. § 2000e(k).

[19] H.R. REP. NO. 95-948, at 3 (1978) (report from the Committee on Education and Labor to accompany the House version of the PDA, H.R. 6075); *see also* S. REP. NO. 95-331, at 3 (1977) (report from the Committee on Human Resources to accompanying the Senate version of the PDA, S. 995) (stating that the measure was "intended to make plain that, under title VII of the Civil Rights Act of 1964, discrimination based on pregnancy,

The PDA's legislative history also suggests that, in enacting the statute, Congress did not mean to single out pregnant women for special protection.[20] On the other hand, the PDA's requirement that pregnant women "be treated the same . . . as other persons not so affected but similar in their ability or inability to work" is unlike safeguards Title VII provides other protected groups; the statute does not use similar language elsewhere.[21] This unique language has caused some confusion in the courts—most notably in assessing claims alleging disparate impact (claims that a neutral action has an unjustified discriminatory effect).[22] The language in the second phrase has also led to confusion about whether being treated "the same" means that pregnant women must receive accommodations given other workers for nonpregnancy reasons,[23] although accommodations claims in the future may be resolved under the PWFA as discussed below.[24]

Certain pregnant employees additionally fall outside the PDA's protections. Title VII incorporates some exemptions, and these apply to the PDA. For instance, the statute does not cover employers of fewer than 15 workers.[25] Other categories of employers, including military servicemembers and most federal judicial employers, fall outside Title VII's purview.[26] Title

---

childbirth, and related medical conditions is discrimination based on sex"); *Newport News*, 462 U.S. at 681 (discussing legislative history of PDA).

[20] S. REP. NO. 95-331, at 4 ("Basic to all of these applications is that the bill, because it would operate as part of title VII, prohibits only discriminatory treatment. Therefore, the bill does not require employers to treat pregnant women in any particular manner with respect to hiring, permitting them to continue working, providing sick leave, furnishing medical and hospital benefits, providing disability benefits, or any other matter. The bill would simply require that pregnant women be treated the same as other employees on the basis of their ability or inability to work."); H.R. REP. NO. 95-948, at 3–4 ("We recognize that enactment of [the House version of the PDA] will reflect no new legislative mandate of the congress nor effect changes in practices, costs, or benefits beyond those intended by Title VII of the Civil Rights Act. On the contrary, the narrow approach utilized by the bill is to eradicate confusion by expressly broadening the definition of sex discrimination in Title VII to include pregnancy-based discrimination.").

[21] 42 U.S.C. § 2000e(k); *see also* Young v. United Parcel Serv., Inc., 575 U.S. 206, 219 (2015) (noting "the meaning of the second clause is less clear" than that of the first clause).

[22] For a discussion of this textual difference in the disparate impact context, see *infra* notes 132–139 and accompanying text.

[23] *See infra* notes 78–130 and accompanying text.

[24] *See infra* notes 165–192 and accompanying text.

[25] 42 U.S.C. § 2000e(b); U.S. EQUAL EMP. OPPORTUNITY COMM'N, PREGNANCY DISCRIMINATION AND PREGNANCY-RELATED DISABILITY DISCRIMINA TION, https://www.eeoc.gov/pregnancy-discrimination (last visited June 7, 2023).

[26] 42 U.S.C. §§ 2000e(f), 2000e-16(a) ("applying protections to "units of the judicial branch of the Federal Government having positions in the competitive service"); Frost v. United States, 115 Fed. Cl. 252, 256 (2014)(observing that "the only units in the judicial branch that have ever had positions in the competitive service are the Administrative Office of the

VII also allows religious institutions more leeway than others to make employment decisions.[27]

Elements of a PDA Claim: Adverse Action and Motive

Under the PDA, plaintiffs may raise claims like those under Title VII's other protected bases, including claims based on harassment or adverse action based on pregnancy. They may also raise a PDA-specific claim—that the employer did not accommodate pregnant women as it did others similarly situated. For an adverse action claim, proving a PDA violation generally requires showing two primary elements: an adverse employment action and discriminatory motivation.[28] On the first, Title VII, and therefore the PDA, prohibits discrimination in the "compensation, terms, conditions, or privileges of employment."[29] An adverse employment action is one such as termination, discipline, or loss of pay that is significant enough to change the terms, conditions, or privileges of employment.[30] Other examples of adverse

United States Courts and the Federal Judicial Center" and, accordingly, federal judiciary employees "do not generally qualify as competitive service employees because they are neither in the executive branch nor included in the competitive service by statute."); Jackson v. Modly, 949 F.3d 763, 772 (D.C. Cir. 2020) (noting every circuit to have considered the issue has concluded, although not always for the same reasons, that Title VII applies only to civilian Department of Defense employees, not uniformed servicemembers); 29 C.F.R. § 1614.103(d)(1) (noting Title VII regulations do not apply to "[u]niformed members of the military departments").

[27] 42 U.S.C. § 2000e-1(a) (indicating religious institutions may employ "individuals of a particular religion to perform work connected with the carrying on . . . of [their] activities"); *see also id.* § 2000e-2(e)(2). The Constitution also constrains some employment laws. As interpreted by the Supreme Court, the Constitution provides a "ministerial exception" forbidding regulation of religious institutions' selection and management of leaders and others performing religious functions. Hosanna-Tabor Evangelical Lutheran Church & Sch. v. EEOC, 565 U.S. 171, 188, 196 (2012) (holding ministerial exception limits religious teacher's entitlement to ADA protections and noting lower courts' application of the doctrine to Title VII claims); Our Lady of Guadalupe Sch. v. Morrissey-Berru, 140 S. Ct. 2049, 2066 (2020) (holding ministerial exception applies to primary school teachers at Catholic schools to bar age and disability discrimination claims). See also Cong. Rsch. Serv., *Church Leadership and the Ministerial Exception*, *Constitution Annotated*, https://constitution.congress.gov/browse/essay/amdt1-2-3-4/ALDE_00013117/['ministerial'] (last visited June 21, 2023).

[28] Claims based on a disparate impact theory or a failure to treat pregnant workers the same as those similarly situated have different intent requirements; these will be discussed separately.

[29] 42 U.S.C. § 2000e-2(a)(1).

[30] EEOC ENFORCEMENT GUIDANCE, *supra* note 2; Asmo v. Keane, Inc., 471 F.3d 588, 592 (6th Cir. 2006).

employment actions that often arise in the PDA context include involuntary reassignment or leave, including mandatory light duty when the employee did not request or require it.[31]

In many cases, the parties agree that the employee has faced an adverse employment action, such as failure to be hired, discharge, threat of discharge, or promotion denial, and the case turns on the second element: whether the employer acted because of the employee's pregnancy.[32] In considering whether an employer mistreated an employee "because of" pregnancy, federal courts generally apply the same legal standards they would in a sex or race discrimination case. In determining motive, courts may consider any unfavorable comments made by supervisors about an employee's pregnancy. Plaintiffs have recounted statements about a worker's appearance, disapproval of her pregnancy, or disparagement of her working ability. Alleged comments noted in PDA cases include "take your fat pregnant ass home,"[33] "[y]ou picked a poor time to get pregnant,"[34] or, to a recently married employee, "we feared something like this would happen."[35] One manager allegedly told a pregnant worker "if she wanted to keep her job, she should not stay pregnant."[36] Such statements may support the employee's claim that an employer acted with a discriminatory motive.

If courts do not find direct evidence of antipregnancy bias, they will turn to the burden-shifting framework announced in *McDonnell Douglas Corp. v. Green*.[37] A PDA plaintiff must show that an employer knew of her pregnancy

---

[31] Richards v. City of Topeka, 173 F.3d 1247, 1250 (10th Cir. 1999); Carney v. Martin Luther Home, Inc., 824 F.2d 643, 648 (8th Cir. 1987); *see also* S. REP. NO. 95-331 at 3–4 (1978) (report from the Committee on Human Resources to accompany the Senate version of the PDA, S. 995) (stating that when pregnant employees are "not able to work for medical reasons, they must be accorded the same rights, leave privileges and other benefits, as other workers who are disabled from working").

[32] Germain v. Cnty. of Suffolk, No. 07-CV-2523-ADS ARL, 2009 WL 1514513, at *6 (E.D.N.Y. May 29, 2009); Poague v. Huntsville Wholesale Furniture, No. 7:18-CV-00005-LSC, 2020 WL 6363983, at *3 (N.D. Ala. Oct. 29, 2020).

[33] Hercule v. Wendy's of N.E. Fla., Inc., No. 10-80248-CIV, 2010 WL 1882181, at *1 (S.D. Fla. May 11, 2010) (recounting facts in granting partial motion to dismiss against improper parties).

[34] Villanueva v. Christiana Care Health Servs., Inc., No. CIV.A. 04-258-JJF, 2007 WL 188111, at *2 (D. Del. Jan. 23, 2007) (denying motion for summary judgment, holding alleged comments provided circumstantial evidence of discriminatory termination).

[35] Hamilton v. Southland Christian Sch., Inc., 680 F.3d 1316, 1320 (11th Cir. 2012) (holding alleged statements provided circumstantial evidence of discriminatory motive for termination, precluding summary judgment for employer), *overruled in part by* United States v. Durham, 795 F.3d 1329, 1330 (11th Cir. 2015).

[36] Townsend v. Town of Brusly, 421 F. Supp. 3d 352, 360 (M.D. La. 2019).

[37] 411 U.S. 792, 802–04 (1973).

or related condition, prove that she satisfactorily performed her job (or was qualified for hire or promotion), identify an adverse employment action, and point to circumstances suggesting the employer acted because of pregnancy.[38]

Courts can consider any workplace circumstances that would support an inference of discrimination. Such circumstances may include more favorable treatment of a similarly situated worker who is not pregnant. For example, the U.S. Court of Appeals for the Sixth Circuit held that, for an employee allegedly disciplined and fired one month after disclosing her pregnancy, "the sequence of events . . . is sufficient to raise the inference of discrimination."[39] As in other discrimination cases, courts may infer discrimination when employers fail to give credible, consistent reasons for the adverse action.[40] An employer may lack credibility, for example, when managers' given reasons for firing a pregnant employee change after she files suit.[41] Changing standards after an employee announces a pregnancy can also signal discrimination. One employer at an auto-parts store, for example, allegedly decided on the position's lifting requirement only *after* a worker became pregnant. In setting the lifting requirement, the plaintiff claimed that the manager said: "'what was the weight I told you?' then, after some indecision, decid[ed] that she must lift 50 pounds, and finally conclud[ed] 'oh well, I guess you don't meet it. So you can't come back to work.'"[42]

Once a worker or applicant has presented facts supporting an inference of discrimination, the burden shifts to the employer to produce evidence that it had a "legitimate, nondiscriminatory reason" for its action.[43] If the employer can produce such evidence, the burden shifts back to the employee to prove that the proffered reason is pretextual—i.e., that the real motive was pregnancy.[44] The employee may prevail even if there were multiple motives—both a discriminatory motive and a legitimate one. It is enough if pregnancy

---

[38] *See* Lewis v. City of Union City, 918 F.3d 1213, 1221 (11th Cir. 2019).

[39] Lenzi v. Systemax, Inc., 944 F.3d 97, 108 (2d Cir. 2019); *see also* Asmo v. Keane, Inc., 471 F.3d 588, 594 (6th Cir. 2006) (holding two-month window "sufficient to establish a link between [employee's] pregnancy and her termination").

[40] Legg v. Ulster Cnty., 820 F.3d 67, 70 (2d Cir. 2016).

[41] *Asmo*, 471 F.3d at 596 (pointing to evidence suggesting inconsistent statement and reversing summary judgment).

[42] Stansfield v. O'Reilly Auto., Inc., No. CIV.A. H-04-4161, 2006 WL 1030010, at *3 (S.D. Tex. Apr. 19, 2006) (denying defendant's summary judgment motion).

[43] *McDonnell Douglas Corp. v. Green*, 411 U.S. 411, 802 (1973); Plotke v. White, 405 F.3d 1092, 1100 (10th Cir.2005).

[44] *McDonnell Douglas*, 411 U.S. at 804; Lewis v. City of Union City, 918 F.3d 1213, 1221 (11th Cir. 2019).

was "a motivating factor" in the adverse decision, even if "other factors also motivated the practice."[45]

Pregnancy-motivated adverse action is discriminatory even if the employer characterizes its decision as protective or benign.[46] As the Supreme Court stated, "stereotypical assumptions" about pregnant workers' abilities "would, of course, be inconsistent with Title VII's goal of equal employment opportunity."[47]

Pregnancy Harassment

In addition to barring adverse actions such as reassignment or termination, Title VII and the PDA make it illegal for an employer to subject an employee to a hostile work environment because of pregnancy.[48] This type of claim requires evidence of "severe or pervasive conduct such that it constitutes a change in the terms and conditions of employment," although the plaintiff need not identify a discrete adverse employment action.[49] The Supreme Court has described a workplace that is "permeated with 'discriminatory intimidation, ridicule, and insult'" as "sufficiently severe or pervasive to alter the conditions of the victim's employment and create an abusive working environment."[50]

A single derogatory comment is rarely enough to show a hostile work environment.[51] It is also not enough that a particular employee found the workplace unwelcoming; a harassment claim requires that an "objectively

---

[45] 42 U.S.C. § 2000e-2(m); *see also* Spees v. James Marine, Inc., 617 F.3d 380, 390 (6th Cir. 2010). A plaintiff's damages may be reduced if an employer can show that, even without the discriminatory motive, it would have taken the same action. 42 U.S.C. § 2000e-5(g)(2)(B); Gudenkauf v. Stauffer Commc'ns, Inc., 158 F.3d 1074, 1076 (10th Cir. 1998).

[46] Int'l Union, United Auto., Aerospace & Agr. Implement Workers of Am., UAW v. Johnson Controls, Inc., 499 U.S. 187, 199 (1991) (holding that barring fertile women from jobs with chemical exposure violates the PDA and stating that "the absence of a malevolent motive does not convert a facially discriminatory policy into a neutral policy with a discriminatory effect").

[47] Cal. Fed. Sav. & Loan Ass'n v. Guerra, 479 U.S. 272, 290 (1987).

[48] Harris v. Forklift Sys., Inc., 510 U.S. 17, 21 (1993); U.S. EQUAL EMP. OPPORTUNITY COMM'N, HARASSMENT, https://www.eeoc.gov/harassment (last visited June 7, 2023).

[49] Gorski v. N.H. Dep't of Corr., 290 F.3d 466, 469 (1st Cir. 2002) (quoting Gorski v. N.H. Dep't of Corr., CIV. 99- 562-JD, 2000 WL 1507428 (D.N.H. July 19, 2000)).

[50] *Harris*, 510 U.S. at 21 (quoting Meritor Savings Bank, FSB v. Vinson, 477 U.S. 57, 65–67 (1986)).

[51] *Cf. Gorski*, 290 F.3d at 474 (holding allegation of seven harassing comments adequate to survive summary judgment).

reasonable person would find" the workplace hostile or abusive.[52] Assessment of the working environment is fact-specific, and courts must examine "the totality of the circumstances."[53] These circumstances may include the frequency of the offensive conduct, its severity, whether it is physically threatening or humiliating, and whether it interferes with job performance.[54] Consideration of all the circumstances means that a court will assess pregnancy-based epithets and mistreatment together with any abuse that is not overtly pregnancy-related, such as closer supervision or excessive discipline.[55]

Pregnancy-related hostile work environment claims often allege disparaging comments or threats. In one case, for example, the plaintiff claimed that a manager "beg[a]n referring to [plaintiff] as 'prego'" and urged her to quit or go on disability.[56] A manager pressuring an employee to terminate her pregnancy may support a hostile work environment claim.[57]

"Related Medical Conditions" and the PDA's Scope

Courts have relied both on the PDA's plain text, specifically the protection it extends to "childbirth" and "related medical conditions,"[58] and its legislative history[59] to establish that the statute covers more than pregnancy per se. As one court put it, discrimination "before, during, and after . . . pregnancy" may violate the PDA.[60] The EEOC has stated that "the PDA covers all aspects of

---

[52] *Id.*

[53] Hyde v. K.B. Home, Inc., 355 F. App'x 266, 272 (11th Cir. 2009); *see also Gorski*, 290 F.3d at 471.

[54] Miller v. Kenworth of Dothan, Inc., 277 F.3d 1269, 1276 (11th Cir. 2002).

[55] Zisumbo v. McCleodUSA Telecomms. Servs., Inc., 154 F. App'x 715, 726 (10th Cir. 2005).

[56] *Id.* (reversing summary judgment granted for employer).

[57] Bergstrom-Ek v. Best Oil Co., 153 F.3d 851, 854–55 (8th Cir. 1998) (discussing plaintiff's allegation that employer told her at least six times to get an abortion, calling her at home and offering to pay for it); Hercule v. Wendy's of N.E. Fla., Inc., No. 10-80248-CIV, 2010 WL 1882181, at *1 (S.D. Fla. May 11, 2010) (describing allegation that manager encouraged plaintiff to have an abortion).

[58] Turic v. Holland Hosp., Inc., 85 F.3d 1211, 1214 (6th Cir. 1996) (holding that the "plain language of the statute" barred discrimination on the basis that a worker had considered an abortion).

[59] Pacourek v. Inland Steel Co., 858 F. Supp. 1393, 1402 (N.D. Ill. 1994) (indicating that PDA coverage for claims from women trying to become pregnant rested on a "common-sense reading of the PDA's language," and finding support in statement from Senator that women historically endured discrimination "[b]ecause of their capacity to become pregnant" and "because they might become pregnant" (quoting 123 Cong. Rec. 29385 (1977) (statement of Sen. Harrison Williams)).

[60] *Id.* at 1402; *see also* Hall v. Nalco Co., 534 F.3d 644, 649 (7th Cir. 2008).

pregnancy and all aspects of employment, including hiring, firing, promotion, health insurance benefits, and treatment."[61]

Pre-pregnancy discrimination can include adverse action taken on account of a woman's plans to start a family or seek fertility treatments. For example, the Seventh Circuit concluded that a worker could bring a PDA claim after her employer allegedly fired her for taking time off for fertility treatments, telling her "that the termination was 'in [her] best interest due to [her] health condition.'"[62] In another case of pre-pregnancy discrimination, a federal district court in Illinois rejected an employer's argument that the PDA did not cover discrimination based on inability to become pregnant naturally.[63] The court held that the PDA protected an employee who alleged that her supervisor "verbally abused [her]" about her fertility treatments, questioned whether she could manage pregnancy and career, and treated her sick leave applications less favorably than other workers' requests.[64]

In a similar vein, employers may not bar women of childbearing age from certain jobs under "fetal protection" policies designed to prevent exposure to toxins linked to birth defects.[65] Such policies violate Title VII's bar on sex-based classifications, the Supreme Court has concluded, and the PDA "bolster[s]" this conclusion.[66]

Courts have also applied the PDA to various postpregnancy conditions. A woman may not be fired because of recent childbirth, for example.[67] Postpartum medical complications are impermissible grounds for adverse employment action as well.[68] As one court put it, the PDA encompasses

---

[61] EEOC ENFORCEMENT GUIDANCE, *supra* note 2.

[62] *Hall*, 534 F.3d at 649 (rejecting district court's conclusion that because infertility is gender-neutral, plaintiff could not pursue a Title VII claim).

[63] *Pacourek*, 858 F. Supp. at 1401; *see also* Batchelor v. Merck & Co., 651 F. Supp. 2d 818, 830 (N.D. Ind. 2008) (holding PDA protects against discrimination based on a woman's plans to become pregnant); Erickson v. Bd. of Governors of State Colleges & Universities for Ne. Ill. Univ., 911 F. Supp. 316, 319 (N.D. Ill. 1995) (holding PDA covers infertility treatment).

[64] *Pacourek*, 858 F. Supp. at 1401. *But see* In re Union Pac. R.R. Emp. Pracs. Litig., 479 F.3d 936, 941 (8th Cir. 2007) (holding medical plan's exclusion of infertility treatment does not violate the PDA because "[i]nfertility is strikingly different from pregnancy" (internal quotation marks omitted)).

[65] Int'l Union, United Auto., Aerospace & Agr. Implement Workers of Am., UAW v. Johnson Controls, Inc., 499 U.S. 187, 193 (1991).

[66] *Id.* at 197–98 (holding battery manufacturer could not preclude women of childbearing age from employment on the grounds that chemical exposure would be dangerous to a fetus should a worker become pregnant); *see also* EEOC ENFORCEMENT GUIDANCE, *supra* note 2.

[67] Neessen v. Arona Corp., 708 F. Supp. 2d 841, 851 (N.D. Iowa 2010); Shafrir v. Ass'n of Reform Zionists of Am., 998 F. Supp. 355, 363 (S.D.N.Y. 1998).

[68] Reilly v. Revlon, Inc., 620 F. Supp. 2d 524, 544 (S.D.N.Y. 2009).

"conditions related to pregnancy that occur after the actual pregnancy."[69] A woman with a postpartum condition must be treated as are other workers with nonpregnancy illnesses.[70] Courts have held that postpartum depression and a disrupted menstrual cycle, for example, fall within this rule.[71]

Courts have disagreed about whether lactation is a pregnancy-related condition covered by the PDA. At least at first, the prevailing view among reviewing district courts was that breastfeeding was ineligible for PDA protection, as it was viewed as a medical condition related not to pregnancy or childbirth but instead to subsequent child care.[72] At least two federal courts of appeals have also opined, either in a holding or in nonbinding dicta, that breastfeeding is not a protected medical condition under the PDA.[73] However, more recent court decisions, including one by a federal court of appeals, have concluded otherwise,[74] leading one district court in 2016 to identify a "trend" by reviewing courts to "hold that lactation is a 'condition related to

---

[69] *Id.*

[70] *Id.* at 545.

[71] *Id.* at 544 (holding PDA covers postpartum depression); Harper v. Thiokol Chem. Corp., 619 F.2d 489, 493 (5th Cir. 1980) (holding employer's policy of denying postpregnancy employment until worker had returned to a normal menstrual cycle violated PDA); *see also* Infante v. Ambac Fin. Grp., No. 03 CV 8880, 2006 WL 44172, at *4 (S.D.N.Y. Jan. 5, 2006) (noting that plaintiff's thyroid condition, if exacerbated by recent pregnancy, might fall within the PDA's purview), *aff'd*, 257 F. App'x 432 (2d Cir. 2007).

[72] *See, e.g.*, Fejes v. Gilpin Ventures, Inc., 960 F. Supp. 1487, 1491 (D. Colo. 1997) (observing that reviewing courts had "uniformly held that needs or conditions of the child which require the mother's presence are not within the scope of the PDA"); Jacobson v. Regent Assisted Living, Inc., No. CV-98-564-ST, 1999 WL 373790, at *11 (D. Or. Apr. 9, 1999); Wallace v. Pyro Mining Co., 789 F. Supp. 867, 869–70 (W.D. Ky. 1990) (examining the text and legislative history of the PDA and stating that "[w]hile it may be that breast-feeding and weaning are natural concomitants of pregnancy and childbirth, they are not 'medical conditions' related thereto Nothing in the Pregnancy Discrimination Act, or Title VII, obliges employers to accommodate the child-care concerns of breast-feeding female workers by providing additional breast-feeding leave not available to male workers"), *aff'd*, 951 F.2d 351 (6th Cir. 1991).

[73] Derungs v. Wal-Mart Stores, Inc., 374 F.3d 428, 438 (6th Cir. 2004) (assessing state law claim and suggesting in dicta that the PDA would not reach breastfeeding); Wallace v. Pyro Min. Co., 951 F.2d 351, (No. 90–6259, 1991 WL 270823, at *1 (6th Cir. Dec. 19, 1991)) (per curiam) (table, text in Westlaw) (stating in dicta that the PDA would not cover breastfeeding); Notter v. N. Hand Prot., a Div. of Siebe, Inc., 89 F.3d 829, 1996 WL 342008, at *5 (4th Cir. June 21, 1996) (table, text in Westlaw) (describing aspects of Fourth Circuit's prior ruling in *Barrash v. Bowen*, 846 F.2d 927, 931 (4th Cir. 1988) (per curiam), about the scope of the PDA as "dicta without any citation of authority," but maintaining that the earlier case "stands for the narrow proposition that breastfeeding is not a *medical* condition related to pregnancy or to childbirth").

[74] EEOC v. Houston Funding II, Ltd., 717 F.3d 425, 428 (5th Cir. 2013); Hicks v. City of Tuscaloosa, 870 F.3d 1253, 1258–59 (11th Cir. 2017); Allen-Brown v. District of Columbia, 174 F. Supp. 3d 463, 479 (D.D.C. 2016).

pregnancy'" under the PDA.[75] Courts taking this view have emphasized, for example, that a woman unable to breastfeed may experience pain, infection, or other medical complications.[76] Since 2010, nursing mothers have also enjoyed additional statutory protections: as discussed below, the Fair Labor Standards Act mandates breaks for covered nursing mothers.[77]

Pregnancy Accommodation and *Young v. United Parcel Service*

At its core, the PDA calls for pregnant workers to be treated the same as other similarly situated employees.[78] After the PDA's passage, courts struggled to decide which workers were similarly situated under the Act. Pregnant women often face work restrictions, such as lifting constraints, limits on chemical exposure, a need for more bathroom breaks, or other scheduling requirements that need accommodating.[79]

The PDA does not forbid employers from granting accommodations for such constraints, but it does not require accommodations for pregnant workers—at least in circumstances where accommodations are not offered to others.[80] The difficulty in applying the PDA comes when an employer offers accommodation to some nonpregnant workers and not to pregnant workers. Then PDA plaintiffs may bring claims based on the denial of accommodations and produce evidence of comparators—nonpregnant workers who, they allege, are similarly situated and were treated more favorably. Courts at first varied in their approach to evaluating comparators. Some courts concluded that the reason an employee needed an accommodation mattered, holding that

---

[75] *Hicks*, 870 F.3d at 1259 n.5 (quoting Mayer v. Pro. Ambulance, LLC, 211 F. Supp. 3d 408, 417 (D.R.I. 2016)).

[76] *Allen-Brown*, 174 F. Supp. 3d at 479; *see also Mayer*, 211 F. Supp. 3d at 417.

[77] Fair Labor Standards Act, 29 U.S.C. §§ 207(r), 218c (as amended by the Providing Urgent Maternal Protections for Nursing Mothers Act, Pub. L. No. 117-328, Div. KK, 136 Stat. 4459 (2022) [hereinafter PUMP for Nursing Mothers Act]; *see infra* notes 197–207 and accompanying text.

[78] 42 U.S.C. § 2000e(k).

[79] Bradley A. Areheart, *Accommodating Pregnancy*, 67 ALA. L. REV. 1125, 1133 (2016) ("The most commonly requested accommodations include frequent bathroom breaks, limits on heavy lifting, and limitations on overtime work."); Jackson v. J.R. Simplot Co., 666 F. App'x 739, 740 (10th Cir. 2016) (unpublished, nonprecedential opinion recognizing employee's doctor restricted her exposure to three chemicals present at her workplace).

[80] Cal. Fed. Sav. & Loan Ass'n v. Guerra, 479 U.S. 272, 285 (1987) (indicating "Congress intended the PDA to be a floor beneath which pregnancy disability benefits may not drop—not a ceiling above which they may not rise" (internal quotation marks and citation omitted)).

employers must treat pregnant women the same as employees with off-the-job injuries, but that employees injured on the job were not relevant comparators.[81] Other courts concluded that any accommodated employees were relevant.[82] As the Sixth Circuit reasoned, because the PDA's text references only employees' "ability to work," and not any other basis for comparison, an employer who accommodated on-the-job injuries must accommodate pregnant workers with similar restrictions.[83]

The Supreme Court addressed the issue in its 2015 decision in *Young v. United Parcel Service*,[84] clarifying that employers must provide accommodations for pregnant women only in limited situations.[85] In the Court's view, employers could rely on circumstances beyond employees' physical needs to justify disparate treatment. Following *Young*, federal courts have wrestled with its application to workers' claims that, when it comes to pregnancy accommodations, they have been treated less favorably than other employees similar in their ability to work.

The Young Decision

In Young, the Supreme Court considered a United Parcel Service (UPS) delivery driver's request for light duty. Young requested light duty after she became pregnant and her doctor restricted her from heavy lifting. UPS denied her request, even though it offered light duty to some other groups of workers, including those who were injured on the job, those who lost Department of Transportation licensure, or those who had disabilities recognized under the Americans with Disabilities Act (ADA). Young claimed pregnancy discrimination, asserting that UPS's refusal to extend the same privilege to pregnant employees who were similar in their ability to work violated the PDA.[86]

---

[81] Serednyj v. Beverly Healthcare, LLC, 656 F.3d 540, 548–49 (7th Cir. 2011) (holding no PDA violation where employer accommodated employees injured on the job and those entitled under the ADA but not pregnant workers), *abrogated by* Young v. United Parcel Serv., Inc., 575 U.S. 206 (2015); Spivey v. Beverly Enterprises, Inc., 196 F.3d 1309, 1313 (11th Cir. 1999) (holding employees injured on the job are not comparable to pregnant workers for PDA purposes), *abrogated by Young*, 575 U.S. at 206.

[82] Ensley-Gaines v. Runyon, 100 F.3d 1220, 1226 (6th Cir. 1996) *abrogated by Young*, 575 U.S. at 206; *see also* EEOC v. Horizon/CMS Healthcare Corp., 220 F.3d 1184, 1196 (10th Cir. 2000).

[83] *Ensley-Gaines*, 100 F.3d at 1226.

[84] 575 U.S. 206 (2015).

[85] *Id.* at 206.

[86] Young v. United Parcel Serv., Inc., 575 U.S. 206, 211–15 (2015).

The Supreme Court agreed that the PDA requires a court to compare accommodations given pregnant and nonpregnant workers to implement the statute's requirement that pregnant workers be treated as favorably as others similar in their ability to work. In the Court's view, the PDA entails more than "[s]imply including pregnancy among Title VII's protected traits," and thereby barring adverse employment actions based on pregnancy, because that approach "would not overturn Gilbert in full."[87] The PDA's second phrase—that "women affected by pregnancy, childbirth, or related medical conditions shall be treated the same for all employment-related purposes . . . as other persons not so affected but similar in their ability or inability to work"[88]—would be rendered "superfluous" if the statute did not require employers to accommodate pregnant employees in at least some situations when they accommodated others.[89]

In a six-to-three decision (with Justice Alito concurring), however, the Court ultimately recognized only a narrow accommodation requirement. The Court held that determining when employees are "similar in their ability or inability to work," and therefore whether employers must make workplace adjustments for pregnant workers, depends not just on whether an employer accommodates other workers, but why it does so. To allow a pregnant employee to point to any accommodation of another worker to entitle her to light duty, the Court held, would be to grant a sort of "most-favored-nation" status to pregnant women that the PDA did not require.[90] It would be too much, the Court reasoned, if "[a]s long as an employer provides one or two workers with an accommodation—say, those with particularly hazardous jobs, or those whose workplace presence is particularly needed, or those who have worked at the company for many years, or those who are over the age of 55—then it must provide similar accommodations to all pregnant workers."[91]

Turning to the facts of the case before it, the Court determined that although UPS granted various accommodations, the record did not show whether other workers were truly "similar in their ability or inability to work" within the Court's understanding of the PDA.[92]

---

[87] *Id.* at 227.
[88] 42 U.S.C. § 2000e(k).
[89] *Young*, 575 U.S. at 226.
[90] *Id.* at 221.
[91] *Id.*
[92] *Id.* at 229–230; *id.* at 237–41 (Alito, J., concurring) (noting various accommodations UPS had granted, and the lack of explanation for some).

As a result, while Young could rely on other workers' accommodations as evidence of discrimination, the Court held that those accommodations did not necessarily show that she was entitled to a pregnancy accommodation.[93] The employer could still prevail by explaining its sex- neutral reasons for accommodating others. In this case, UPS had unique reasons for offering each type of accommodation.[94] UPS wanted to implement the ADA, to comply with collective bargaining agreements, and to continue to employ workers who—unlike Young—had lost their licensure but not their ability to lift packages.[95] Such reasons, the Court surmised, might show on remand that UPS did not single out pregnant women for exclusion from its accommodation procedures.[96]

Along with an assessment of the employer's reasons for treating pregnant workers less favorably than others, the Court announced one more step in the PDA analysis: a holistic view of an employer's accommodations. According to the Supreme Court, a court should consider "the combined effects of" an employer's policies and decide whether they significantly burden pregnant employees in a way that suggests intentional discrimination. "[E]vidence that the employer accommodates a large percentage of nonpregnant workers while failing to accommodate a large percentage of pregnant employees" would suggest such a burden, the Court opined.[97] A court would then consider "the strength of [the employer's] justifications for each [accommodation] when combined,"[98] and the employer's reasons must be "sufficiently strong" to justify the burden on pregnant workers.[99] If the reasons are not strong enough, the Court held, the circumstances may "give rise to an inference of intentional discrimination."[100] Cost alone, the Court added, would not "normally" meet this test to justify different treatment of pregnant workers.[101] The Court considered this assessment of accommodations "consistent with our longstanding rule that a plaintiff can use circumstantial proof to rebut an employer's apparently legitimate, nondiscriminatory reasons for treating individuals within a protected class differently than those outside the protected

[93] *Id.* at 229.
[94] *Id.* at 218–21.
[95] *Id.* at 215–16, 218.
[96] *Id.* at 232.
[97] *Id* at 229.
[98] *Id.* at 231.
[99] *Id.* at 229.
[100] *Id.*
[101] *Id.* at 229.

class."[102] With these principles in place, the Court remanded Young's case to the Fourth Circuit.[103]

Justice Alito, concurring in the judgment, agreed that a rule only prohibiting adverse employment actions based on pregnancy would render superfluous the second phrase of the PDA, which "raises several difficult questions of interpretation."[104] In Justice Alito's view, the PDA required only a limited assessment of comparators—those doing identical or very similar work.[105] In support of this constrained view of accommodations, Justice Alito pointed out that the PDA does not use the broad language that the ADA and Title VII's protections for religious practice employ, both of which explicitly require some "accommodation" unless it would impose an "undue hardship."[106]

In dissent, Justice Scalia, joined by Justices Kennedy and Thomas, concluded that the PDA did not offer pregnant workers protection exceeding that of other protected classes.[107] In amending Title VII, Congress simply made clear that pregnancy discrimination is sex discrimination, in Justice Scalia's view.[108] Under this reading, an employer need not offer pregnant workers the accommodations offered for injury, because injury is different from pregnancy. Scalia would not have required any holistic analysis of an employer's accommodation rules and their burden on pregnant employees. According to Justice Scalia, an employer simply may not "single[] pregnancy out for disfavor" as did the benefits plan in Gilbert.[109] The PDA's second phrase served to add, in Justice Scalia's judgment, "clarity," not a new substantive protection.[110] In a separate dissent, Justice Kennedy also pointed out that at UPS "[m]any other workers with health- related restrictions were not accommodated either."[111]

Lower Courts' Application of Young

Under the PDA, plaintiffs may raise both a "traditional" Title VII claim (such as harassment or adverse action against a pregnant person with a

---

[102] *Id.* at 230.
[103] *Id.* at 232.
[104] *Id.* at 233 (Alito, J., concurring).
[105] *Id.* at 234 (Alito, J., concurring).
[106] *Id.* at 238 (Alito, J., concurring).
[107] *Id.* at 244 (Scalia, J., dissenting, joined by Kennedy and Thomas, JJ.).
[108] *Id.* (Scalia, J., dissenting).
[109] *Id.*at 246 (Scalia, J., dissenting).
[110] *Id.* at 245 (Scalia, J., dissenting).
[111] *Id.* at 251 (Kennedy, J., dissenting).

discriminatory motive) and a PDA-specific claim (that the employer did not accommodate pregnant women as it did others similarly situated).[112] Young expounded on a test for the second type of claim, requiring courts to evaluate whether accommodation policies excluding pregnant workers "impose a significant burden on pregnant workers" and whether the "legitimate, nondiscriminatory reasons" for the policies are "sufficiently strong to justify the burden."[113] This second type of claim has proven difficult to adjudicate.[114] What is clear from *Young* is that employers may offer light duty or other work modifications to some workers and exclude pregnant workers from those accommodations, but the exclusion must be justified.[115] Otherwise, *Young* does not provide a hard-and-fast rule for assessing pregnancy accommodations. As one Eleventh Circuit judge pointed out, the Supreme Court's decision left "gaps . . . in our understanding of how trial courts should proceed in PDA cases" once there is a preliminary showing of different treatment.[116]

Part of the difficulty arises from the complex facts in *Young*. Young pointed to many, dissimilar workers whom UPS accommodated, including some accommodated because of non-PDA legal obligations and others (such as those who lost licensure) accommodated for unknown reasons.[117] As a result, lower courts applying *Young* have struggled to determine which accommodation circumstances matter in the PDA context.[118] The ultimate

---

[112] 42 U.S.C. § 2000e(k); Allen-Brown v. District of Columbia, 174 F. Supp. 3d 463, 475 (D.D.C. 2016).

[113] *Young*, 575 U.S. at 229 (internal quotation marks omitted); *see also Allen-Brown*, 174 F. Supp. 3d at 475–77 (applying *Young*).

[114] One commentator, stating that *Young*'s "holding is complicated and not perfectly clear," indicated that employers may be inclined to voluntarily extend pregnancy accommodations in order to be "safe rather than sorry." Areheart, *supra* note 79, at 1128 n.7.

[115] *Young*, 575 U.S. at 229.

[116] Durham v. Rural/Metro Corp., 955 F.3d 1279, 1288 (11th Cir. 2020) (Boggs, J., concurring). Business leaders, too, have noted that employers "face great uncertainty" about pregnancy accommodations. Chamber of Com. of the U.S.,

U.S. Chamber Key Vote Letter on the Pregnant Workers Fairness Act (Sept. 14, 2020), https://www.uschamber.com/letters-congress/us-chamber-key-vote-letter-the-pregnant-workers-fairness-act (last visited June 7, 2023).

[117] *Durham*, 955 F.3d at 1288 (Boggs, J., concurring); Lewis v. City of Union City, 918 F.3d 1213, 1228 n.14 (11th Cir. 2019) (noting *Young* identified seven types of accommodated workers, including some accommodated because of other laws or collective bargaining agreements).

[118] *Durham*, 955 F.3d at 1288 (Boggs, J., concurring). One commenter concluded that, under *Young*, employers who accommodate some employees and exclude pregnant employees face "substantial liability risk." Sara Alexander, *Labor Pains: The Inadequacies of Current Federal Pregnancy Laws and the Alternative Routes to Accommodation*, 37 MISS. C. L. REV. 152, 171 (2019).

inquiry, however, remains the question of "whether the employer's actions g[i]ve rise to [a] valid inference of unlawful discrimination."[119]

At the very least, *Young* made it harder for pregnant workers to prevail under the PDA on a claim that they should be accommodated because other workers are accommodated. *Young* overturned the rule, once applied in some courts, that pregnant workers could show discrimination by simply identifying other employees receiving accommodations as comparators.[120] Instead, as the Second Circuit stated, "[w]hether it is appropriate to infer a discriminatory intent from the pattern of exceptions in a particular workplace will depend on the inferences that can be drawn from that pattern and the credibility of the employer's purported reasons for adopting them."[121]

Post-*Young*, some pregnant workers have still managed to raise an inference of discrimination based on the denial of accommodations granted to other workers. For example, a D.C. district court held that a police officer had raised an inference of discrimination when her department awarded light duty to 11 other officers but refused her request for light duty after she found it too painful to wear a bulletproof vest while breastfeeding.[122]

For the most part, applying *Young*, courts require pregnant workers to identify a very similar situation when the employer accommodated a nonpregnant worker before they will infer discrimination against a pregnant worker. One factor courts have considered is whether employees' accommodation needs derive from on-the-job versus off-the-job sources. For example, the Eleventh Circuit considered the case of an emergency medical technician whose pregnancy imposed lifting restrictions.[123] The lower court had concluded that employees accommodated for on-the-job injuries were comparable, but the Eleventh Circuit remanded the case so that the lower court could consider the employer's claimed reasons for treating on-the-job injury and pregnancy differently.[124] Similarly, the Seventh Circuit concluded that a retailer who offered light duty only for on-the-job injuries did not violate the

---

[119] *Durham*, 955 F.3d at 1289 (Boggs, J., concurring) (internal quotation marks and citation omitted).

[120] Young v. United Parcel Serv., Inc., 575 U.S. 206, 210 (2015); Ensley-Gaines v. Runyon, 100 F.3d 1220, 1226 (6th Cir. 1996); *see also* EEOC v. Horizon/CMS Healthcare Corp., 220 F.3d 1184, 1196 (10th Cir. 2000).

[121] Legg v. Ulster Cnty., 820 F.3d 67, 78 (2d Cir. 2016).

[122] Allen-Brown v. District of Columbia, 174 F. Supp. 3d 463, 477 (D.D.C. 2016); *see also Legg*, 820 F.3d at 70–78.

[123] Durham v. Rural/Metro Corp., 955 F.3d 1279, 1282–83 (11th Cir. 2020).

[124] *Id.* at 1283, 1287.

PDA in denying light duty for pregnant workers.[125] These cases reflect that even after pregnant workers identify comparable employees who were granted accommodations, courts may permit employers to justify treating the pregnant workers differently under the PDA. The Second Circuit surmised, for example, that an employer's cited reason for accommodating nonpregnant employees—compliance with state- law requirements for workers injured on the job—might (if true) justify a disparity.[126]

Courts have also looked at whether comparators have similar medical restrictions. For instance, in an unpublished, nonprecedential opinion, the Tenth Circuit declined to find that an employer discriminated against a plaintiff when it gave other workers (and, for a time, the plaintiff) light duty because of lifting restrictions but then denied light duty when the plaintiff's doctor restricted her exposure to chemicals.[127] A proper comparator would be someone needing an accommodation because of chemical restrictions, the Tenth Circuit held, rather than someone with different medical needs.[128]

In some cases, there may be no accommodated employees for comparison. All in all, when an employer never (or hardly ever) grants accommodations for nonpregnant employees, it generally does not have to accommodate a pregnant employee under the PDA.[129] For example, shortly after Young, the Fifth Circuit held in an unpublished, nonprecedential opinion that a nurse fired because of pregnancy-related lifting restrictions could not make out a PDA claim given that the employer accommodated no other nurses with lifting restrictions.[130]

---

[125] Equal Emp. Opportunity Comm'n v. Wal-Mart Stores E., L.P., 46 F.4th 587, 597 (7th Cir. 2022). The court found it significant that the retailer consistently denied light duty requests for all other employees, save those injured at work.

[126] *Legg*, 820 F.3d at 75–78.

[127] Jackson v. J.R. Simplot Co., 666 F. App'x 739, 743 (10th Cir. 2016).

[128] *Id.*; *see also* Santos v. Wincor Nixdorf, Inc., 778 F. App'x 300, 303–04 (5th Cir. 2019) (concluding that employee did not identify a comparator when she could point to no other workers who required telework).

[129] *See, e.g.*, Luke v. CPlace Forest Park SNF, L.L.C., 747 F. App'x 978, 980 (5th Cir. 2019) (per curiam); Durham v. Rural/Metro Corp., No. 4:16-CV-01604-ACA, 2020 WL 7024892, at *4 (N.D. Ala. Nov. 30, 2020); Everett v. Grady Mem'l Hosp. Corp., 703 F. App'x 938, 948 (11th Cir. 2017); Lawson v. City of Pleasant Grove, No. 2:14-CV-0536- JEO, 2016 WL 2338560, at *10 (N.D. Ala. Feb. 16, 2016), *report and recommendation adopted*, No. 2:14-CV-536- KOB, 2016 WL 1719667 (N.D. Ala. Apr. 29, 2016).

[130] *Luke*, 747 F. App'x at 980.

Pregnancy and Disparate Impact Under Title VII

One type of Title VII claim alleges disparate treatment—that an employee suffered adverse action or harassment because of a protected characteristic.[131] Title VII also permits disparate impact claims. In this type of claim, workers challenge a facially neutral employment practice, alleging that it has a disproportionate effect on one group and cannot be justified by business necessity.[132]

A disparate impact claimant does not have to show that an employer intended to single anyone out based on a protected characteristic such as race or sex.

Before the PDA overruled Gilbert and set up special provisions for pregnancy, the Supreme Court had stated in nonbinding dicta that pregnant women could bring disparate impact claims under Title VII.[133] However, some have argued that the PDA precludes a Title VII disparate impact claim based on pregnancy because it requires that a pregnant worker be treated the same as others.[134] Thus, the argument goes, similar treatment cannot be a violation

---

[131] 42 U.S.C. § 2000e-2(a)(1); EEOC ENFORCEMENT GUIDANCE, *supra* note 2; Harris v. Forklift Sys., Inc., 510 U.S. 17, 21 (1993).

[132] Griggs v. Duke Power Co., 401 U.S. 424, 432 (1971); 42 U.S.C. § 2000e-2(k)(1). For further discussion of this theory, see CRS Report R46534, *The Civil Rights Act of 1964: An Overview*, by Christine J. Back, at 72 (2020). A disparate impact theory is distinct from the "significant burden" inquiry announced in *Young v. United Parcel Serv., Inc.*, 575 U.S. 206, 213 (2015), although, in the dissenters' view, the *Young* test risks conflating disparate treatment (i.e., intentional discrimination) with disparate impact (i.e., use of policies with discriminatory effects), 575 U.S. at 249 (Scalia, J., dissenting) (noting "Title VII already has a framework that allows judges to home in on a policy's effects and justifications—disparate impact."); *id.* at 253 (Kennedy, J., dissenting) ("[T]he Court interprets the PDA in a manner that risks conflation of disparate impact with disparate treatment by permitting a plaintiff to use a policy's disproportionate burden on pregnant employees as evidence of pretext." (internal quotation marks omitted)).

[133] Nashville Gas Co. v. Satty, 434 U.S. 136, 144 (1977). The Supreme Court cited precedent establishing a disparate impact theory for claims based on race and stated that "a violation . . . can be established by proof of a discriminatory effect." *Id.* In considering *Gilbert*, the Court suggested that differences in how employee benefits programs treat pregnancy vis-à-vis other medical conditions, in contrast to policies resulting in lesser "employment opportunities or job status" for pregnant workers, would not support a disparate impact claim. *Id.* at 145. The Court ultimately held that a pregnant worker's claim based on sick pay policies must fail under *Gilbert*.

[134] Camille Herbert, *Disparate Impact and Pregnancy: Title VII's Other Accommodation Requirement*, 24 J. GENDER, SOCIAL POLICY & THE LAW 107, 137 (2015); Alexander, *supra* note 118, at 159; Cal. Fed. Sav. & Loan Ass'n v. Guerra, 479 U.S. 272, 298 n.1 (1987) (White, J., dissenting).

even if it has a disparate impact.[135] Still, several courts have considered disparate impact claims under the PDA.[136] The Seventh Circuit emphasized that the PDA is "a definitional amendment" providing "no substantive rule to govern pregnancy discrimination."[137] As such, the court found that the PDA did not eliminate any claims otherwise available under Title VII for pregnancy discrimination. Others also point out that while the Young Court acknowledged the plaintiff had not brought a disparate impact claim, it made no suggestion that such a claim is unavailable for pregnant employees.[138]

EEOC enforcement guidance endorses application of a disparate impact theory to pregnancy discrimination claims. The agency states that while disparate impact claims usually require a statistical showing of the harm of a policy on a protected group, "statistical evidence might not be required if it could be shown that all or substantially all pregnant women would be negatively affected by the challenged policy."[139]

The ADA, Pregnancy-Related Disabilities, and Accommodations

Separate from Title VII and the PDA's protections against certain forms of pregnancy discrimination, the ADA may also provide pregnancy-related protections in some circumstances (although its usefulness may be diminished in the future in light of the Pregnant Workers Fairness Act [PWFA], as discussed below). Title I of the ADA requires that employers reasonably accommodate workers with disabilities.[140] While pregnancy per se is not a disability under the ADA,[141] some women are eligible for protection under the ADA for pregnancy-related disabilities, provided they can perform essential job functions. An ADA-qualifying impairment is one that "substantially limits

---

[135] *Cal. Fed. Sav. & Loan Ass'n*, 479 U.S. at 298 n.1 (White, J., dissenting) ("Whatever remedies Title VII would otherwise provide for victims of disparate impact, Congress expressly ordered pregnancy to be treated in the same manner as other disabilities.").

[136] Smith v. F.W. Morse & Co., 76 F.3d 413, 420–22 (1st Cir. 1996); Scherr v. Woodland Sch. Cmty. Consol. Dist., 867 F.2d 974, 983 (7th Cir. 1988); Germain v. Cnty. of Suffolk, 672 F. Supp. 2d 319, 321 (E.D.N.Y. 2009).

[137] *Scherr*, 867 F.2d at 978.

[138] Young v. United Parcel Serv., Inc., 575 U.S. 206, 213 (2015); Herbert, *supra* note 134, at 138.

[139] EEOC ENFORCEMENT GUIDANCE, *supra* note 2.

[140] 42 U.S.C. § 12112(5).

[141] 29 C.F.R. pt. 1630, app. § 1630.2(h); *Young*, 575 U.S. at 253 (Kennedy, J., dissenting).

one or more" of a person's "major life activities."[142] The Rehabilitation Act creates similar obligations for federally funded programs and most federal employers.[143] The EEOC enforces these provisions.[144] The Congressional Accountability Act applies ADA and Rehabilitation Act standards to legislative employees.[145]

The ADA's application to pregnancy is a recent development in the law.[146] In recent years, courts have applied the ADA to cover postpartum depression,[147] recovery from a caesarian section,[148] lifting restrictions,[149] and pelvic pain.[150] Other complications of pregnancy can include anemia, sciatica, carpal tunnel syndrome, gestational diabetes, nausea with severe dehydration, abnormal heart rhythms, and swelling.[151] These medical conditions can be disabilities under the ADA if they substantially affect major life activities.[152]

Examples of potential ADA accommodations for pregnancy-related disabilities include "allowing a pregnant worker to take more frequent breaks, to keep a water bottle at a work station, or to use a stool; altering how job functions are performed; or providing a temporary assignment to a light duty

---

142 *Young*, 575 U.S. at 218; 42 U.S.C. § 12102(1)(A).

143 29 U.S.C. §§ 791, 794; Khan v. Midwestern Univ., 879 F.3d 838, 843 (7th Cir. 2018), *as amended on denial of reh'g* (Feb. 26, 2018) (applying Rehabilitation Act to medical student claiming pregnancy-related disability).

144 42 U.S.C. § 12117(a); EEOC ENFORCEMENT GUIDANCE, *supra* note 2. The EEOC's Office of Federal Operations enforces Rehabilitation Act provisions for federal employees. U.S. EQUAL EMP. OPPORTUNITY COMM'N, APPEALS, https://www.eeoc.gov/federal-sector/appeals (last visited June 7, 2023).

145 2 U.S.C. 1302(a).

146 Until it was amended in 2008 to expand the statutory definition of "disability," the ADA generally did not protect workers with short-term disabilities, such as those most commonly associated with pregnancy. 42 U.S.C.§ 12102(4)(A); ADA Amendments Act of 2008, Pub. L. No. 110-325, 122 Stat. 3553; Young v. United Parcel Serv., Inc., 575 U.S. 206, 252 (2015) (Kennedy, J., dissenting). The expanded disability coverage from the ADA Amendments Act also applies to Rehabilitation Act claims. Alexander v. Washington Metro. Area Transit Auth., 826 F.3d 544, 547 (D.C. Cir. 2016). Because the plaintiff relied on pre-2008 law, the Supreme Court in the *Young* case did not decide whether the ADA would require the lifting accommodation she requested. *Young*, 575 U.S. at 252 (Kennedy, J., dissenting).

147 Hostettler v. Coll. of Wooster, 895 F.3d 844, 854 (6th Cir. 2018).

148 Price v. UTi, U.S., Inc., No. 4:11-CV-1428 CAS, 2013 WL 798014, at *2–3 (E.D. Mo. Mar. 5, 2013).

149 Heatherly v. Portillo's Hot Dogs, Inc., 958 F. Supp. 2d 913, 921 (N.D. Ill. 2013).

150 McKellips v. Franciscan Health Sys., No. C13-5096MJP, 2013 WL 1991103, at *4 (W.D. Wash. May 13, 2013).

151 U.S. DEP'T OF HEALTH & HUMAN SERVS., OFF. ON WOMEN'S HEALTH, PREGNANCY COMPLICATIONS, https://www.womenshealth.gov/pregnancy/youre-pregnant-now-what/ pregnancy-complications (last visited June 7, 2023).

152 42 U.S.C. § 12102(1)(A); EEOC ENFORCEMENT GUIDANCE, *supra* note 2; *Hostettler*, 895 F.3d at 854.

position."[153] Potential ADA accommodations for pregnancy, like other ADA accommodations, are considered case-by-case, reflecting the worker's impairment and workplace circumstances.

Under the ADA, protected workers first request a workplace change and engage in an "interactive process" with employers to work out a reasonable accommodation.[154] A reasonable accommodation is one that is "feasible," "plausible," and reasonable "in the run of cases."[155] If employers fail to make an accommodation where required, employees may file a complaint with the EEOC and, ultimately, sue in federal court.[156] Employees may seek equitable relief and damages as under Title VII, including, depending on the circumstances, compensatory damages, attorney's fees, and punitive damages.[157]

An employer need not provide an accommodation that imposes an undue hardship on business operations.[158] The ADA requires a case-by-case analysis of the employee's and the employer's circumstances, addressing such factors as the nature and cost of the accommodation, the employer's resources, and the size and function of its workforce.[159] The employer bears the burden of showing an undue hardship, once the employee identifies a reasonable accommodation.[160] Courts have been reluctant to delineate a bright-line rule

---

[153] EEOC ENFORCEMENT GUIDANCE, *supra* note 2.

[154] 29 C.F.R. § 1630.2(o)(3).

[155] US Airways, Inc. v. Barnett, 535 U.S. 391, 401–02 (2002) (holding appropriate accommodation is one that "seems reasonable on its face, *i.e.*, ordinarily or in the run of cases"); Reed v. LePage Bakeries, Inc., 244 F.3d 254, 259 (1st Cir. 2001) (discussing precedent and concluding that "a plaintiff needs to show not only that the proposed accommodation would enable her to perform the essential functions of her job, but also that, at least on the face of things, it is feasible for the employer under the circumstances"); Borkowski v. Valley Cent. Sch. Dist., 63 F.3d 131, 138 (2d Cir. 1995) (holding "it is enough for the plaintiff to suggest the existence of a plausible accommodation").

[156] U.S. EQUAL EMP. OPPORTUNITY COMM'N, FILING A LAWSUIT, https://www.eeoc.gov/filing-lawsuit (last visited June 7, 2023).

[157] 42 U.S.C. §§ 1981, 12205; Kolstad v. Am. Dental Ass'n, 527 U.S. 526, 529, 534 (1999); Bruce v. City of Gainesville, Ga., 177 F.3d 949, 951 (11th Cir. 1999); U.S. EQUAL EMP. OPPORTUNITY COMM'N, REMEDIES FOR EMPLOYMENT DISCRIMINATION, https://www.eeoc.gov/remedies-employment-discrimination (last visited June 7, 2023).

[158] Terrell v. USAir, 132 F.3d 621, 624 (11th Cir. 1998).

[159] 42 U.S.C. § 12111(10)(B); *see* CRS In Focus IF12366, *Reasonable Accommodations for Employees with Disabilities*, by Abigail A. Graber (2023).

[160] LaPorta v. Wal-Mart Stores, Inc., 163 F. Supp. 2d 758, 767 (W.D. Mich. 2001); Severson v. Heartland Woodcraft, Inc., 872 F.3d 476, n.1 480 (7th Cir. 2017) ("The question of undue hardship is a second-tier inquiry under the statute; that is, the hardship exception does not come into play absent a determination that a reasonable accommodation was available.").

regarding what is an undue hardship, producing various outcomes.[161] For example, one district court declined to grant a defendant summary judgment on a pharmacist's request for one day of medical leave, suggesting that whether this was an undue hardship depended on such factors as whether the employer had a replacement pharmacist.[162]

The ADA also excludes some employers and employees from coverage. The statute applies to employers of 15 or more employees, and private clubs and religious employers are afforded certain exemptions.[163] Additionally, going forward, the 2022 PWFA, discussed below, will allow pregnant workers to seek accommodations even without a disability.[164] Because the PWFA allows workers to obtain the same relief they could seek under the ADA, workers may be less likely to invoke the ADA in the future.

The Pregnant Workers Fairness Act

On December 29, 2022, Congress passed the Pregnant Workers Fairness Act as part of the Consolidated Appropriations Act of 2023.[165] The PWFA largely incorporates the accommodation requirements of the ADA, cross-referencing that statute and requiring employers to make "reasonable accommodations" for pregnancy-related limitations.[166] The law is effective June 27, 2023.[167] Some lawmakers supporting the PWFA explained that "varying interpretations [of the PDA and ADA] ha[d] created an unworkable legal framework" and "a lack of clarity" for pregnancy-related accommodations.[168]

---

[161] Nunes v. Wal-Mart Stores, Inc., 164 F.3d 1243, 1247 (9th Cir. 1999); Cleveland v. Fed. Express Corp., 83 F. App'x 74, 78 (6th Cir. 2003); *see also* Dunn v. City of Malden, No. CV 14-14743-RWZ, 2016 WL 10988545, at *4 (D. Mass. Mar. 25, 2016) (stating that dispute of fact existed as to whether plaintiff's request for one additional week of leave unduly burdened employer).

[162] *LaPorta*, 163 F. Supp. 2d at 768; *see also* Jones v. Children's Hosp. of Phila., No. CV 17-5637, 2019 WL 2640060, at *11 (E.D. Pa. June 27, 2019) (applying a state accommodations law requiring the "same framework" as the ADA).

[163] 42 U.S.C. § 12111(5); *see also supra* note 27.

[164] Pregnant Workers Fairness Act, Pub. L. No. 117-328, Division II, § 102(4), 136 Stat. 4459 (2022).

[165] Pub. L. No. 117-328, 136 Stat. 4459 (2022).

[166] *Id.* § 103.

[167] *Id.* § 109; U.S. EQUAL EMP. OPPORTUNITY COMM'N, WHAT YOU SHOULD KNOW ABOUT THE PREGNANT WORKERS FAIRNESS ACT, https://www.eeoc.gov/wysk/what-you-should-know-about-pregnant-workers-fairnessact (last visited June 8, 2023) [hereinafter PWF Act].

[168] H.R. REP. NO. 117-27, at 11 (2021) (Report from the Committee on Education and Labor).

The PWFA mandates "reasonable accommodations" for pregnant workers and gives that term the same construction as in the ADA.[169] In the PWFA's legislative history, lawmakers suggested that reasonable accommodations might include "seating, water, and light duty."[170]

Under the statute's terms and in line with the ADA model, an employer need not provide an accommodation that imposes an undue hardship on business operations.[171] The employer bears the burden of showing an undue hardship, once the employee identifies a reasonable accommodation.[172] As discussed above, ADA case law has not produced bright-line rules in this "fact-specific, individualized inquiry."[173]

As the EEOC regulations require in ADA cases,[174] the PWFA obliges employers and employees to negotiate in good faith to determine appropriate accommodations.[175] The law states that an employee need not accept an accommodation other than one "arrived at through the interactive process."[176] The PWFA also directly addresses mandatory leave, prohibiting employers from forcing employees to take leave if another accommodation would permit them to do their jobs.[177]

The PWFA differs from the ADA in notable ways. While the ADA requires that an employee be able to perform the essential functions of her job,[178] the PWFA protects an employee who cannot perform an essential function if that limitation (1) will be eliminated in the "near future," and (2) can be reasonably accommodated.[179] This provision has come under criticism

---

[169] Pub. L. No. 117-328 § 102(7).

[170] H.R. REP. NO. 117-27, at 11.

[171] Pub. L. No. 117-328, § 102(7) (stating "undue hardship" has the same construction as in the ADA); 42 U.S.C. § 12112(b)(5)(A); Terrell v. USAir, 132 F.3d 621, 624 (11th Cir. 1998).

[172] LaPorta v. Wal-Mart Stores, Inc., 163 F. Supp. 2d 758, 767 (W.D. Mich. 2001); Severson v. Heartland Woodcraft, Inc., 872 F.3d 476, 480 n.1 (7th Cir. 2017).

[173] Nunes v. Wal-Mart Stores, Inc., 164 F.3d 1243, 1247 (9th Cir. 1999); Cleveland v. Fed. Express Corp., 83 F. App'x 74, 78 (6th Cir. 2003); *see also* Dunn v. City of Malden, No. CV 14-14743-RWZ, 2016 WL 10988545, at *4 (D. Mass. Mar. 25, 2016).

[174] 29 C.F.R. § 1630.2(o)(3).

[175] Pub. L. No. 117-328, §§ 102(7), 103(2). An employer who engages in a good faith interactive process gains protection from certain damages. *Id.* § 104(g); *see also* H.R. REP. NO. 117-27, at 34.

[176] Pub. L. No. 117-328, § 103(2); *see* PWF Act, *supra* note 167. Minority views in the House report state that this provision "makes clear reasonable accommodations agreed upon through the interactive process, including an accommodation of leave, are not subject to a unilateral veto by the employee." H.R. REP. NO. 117-27, at 57.

[177] Pub. L. No. 117-328, § 103(4).

[178] 42 U.S.C. §§ 12111(8); 12112(b)(5)(A); 29 C.F.R. § 1630.2(m).

[179] Pub. L. No. 117-328, § 102(6).

from some opponents who suggest that it requires employers to retain a worker who cannot perform fundamental job tasks.[180]

Moreover, under the PWFA, a pregnant worker's impairment need not meet the definition of a "disability" under the ADA before she may claim protection.[181] The PWFA requires accommodations for a "known limitation," which is a "physical or mental condition related to, affected by, or arising out of pregnancy, childbirth, or related medical conditions that the employee or employee's representative has communicated to the employer whether or not such condition meets the definition of disability."[182] Aside from significant congressional guidance through the ADA Amendments Act of 2008, there are regulations and judicial decisions interpreting the ADA's standard for disability.[183] The PWFA standard for a "known limitation" is new, however—how it will play out in practice remains to be seen.[184]

Like the ADA and Title VII, the PWFA applies to employers of 15 or more workers.[185] It protects job applicants, federal workers, and state workers.[186] It covers legislative employees, too, through a cross-reference to the Congressional Accountability Act of 1995.[187] Through cross-reference, it

---

[180] One witness in a committee hearing on a prior version of the bill suggested a worker might "report for work but not do the job." H.R. REP. NO. 116-494, at 51 (2020); *id.* at 53 (quoting labor lawyer Ellen McLaughlin).

[181] Pub. L. No. 117-328, § 102(4).

[182] *Id.*

[183] ADA Amendments Act of 2008, Pub. L. No. 110–325, 122 Stat. 3553; 29 C.F.R. § 1630.2(j)(3); Sugg v. City of Sunrise, No. 20-13884, 2022 WL 4296992, at *8 (11th Cir. Sept. 19, 2022) (acknowledging precedent).

[184] See H.R. REP. NO. 116-494, at 53 (quoting labor lawyer Ellen McLaughlin indicating departure from established ADA standard).

[185] Pub. L. No. 117-328, § 102(2), (3). The statute cross-references Title VII's coverage provisions. Id.; 42 U.S.C.§§ 2000e(b), (f), (n), 2000e-16(a), 2000e-16c(a).

[186] Pub. L. No. 117-328, § 102 (2), (3). The PWFA waives sovereign immunity for state employers. Id. § 106. The Supreme Court has limited the ADA's similar waiver of sovereign immunity, holding that a private individual may not sue a state or state agency for damages for employment discrimination. Board of Trustees of the Univ. of Ala. v. Garrett, 531 U.S. 356 (2001). The Court held that ADA disability protections went beyond Congress's Fourteenth Amendment authority because there was no adequate record showing a pattern of unconstitutional state action discriminating against people with disabilities in employment. Id. at 373. Whether similar challenges to the PWFA may arise remains to be seen.

[187] Pub. L. No. 117-328, § 102(3)(B) (citing 2 U.S.C. § 1301); see PWF Act, supra note 167 ("'Covered employers' include private and public sector employers with at least 15 employees, Congress, Federal agencies, employment agencies, and labor organizations.").

also incorporates the limited applicability of Title VII to religious employers.[188]

The PWFA additionally parallels Title VII for its remedies and enforcement provisions. Remedies could include compensatory damages, punitive damages, and attorneys' fees.[189] Like Title VII and many other antidiscrimination measures, the PWFA bars retaliation against a worker who has requested an accommodation.[190] The law grants the EEOC and the Attorney General enforcement authority as under Title VII and charges the EEOC with issuing regulations, directing it to include examples of reasonable accommodations.[191]

All in all, the PWFA significantly expands employers' obligations to provide needed job modifications to pregnant women. Unlike the ADA, it requires provisional job changes to workers' essential duties, at least in some cases, provided those changes are temporary. It also decouples pregnancy-related accommodation claims from the equal-treatment regime established by the PDA and Title VII. That said, the PWFA applies only to accommodation claims. For claims that an employer discriminated against pregnant workers in other ways, workers must continue to rely on Title VII, state laws, or other applicable laws.[192]

Other Federal Protections for Pregnant Workers

While the PDA, ADA, and PWFA address certain forms of discrimination based on pregnancy and require accommodations in some circumstances, at least three other federal laws also provide pregnancy-related protections. These protections generally involve leave or break time.

---

[188] Pub. L. No. 117-328, § 107(b). This provision exempts "a religious corporation, association, educational institution, or society with respect to the employment of individuals of a particular religion to perform work connected with the carrying on by such corporation, association, educational institution, or society of its activities." 42 U.S.C. § 2000e-1.

[189] Pub. L. No. 117-328, § 104; *see also* H.R. REP. NO. 117-27, at 26 ("[T]he PWFA is written to mirror the enforcement powers, procedures, and remedies established under the Civil Rights Act of 1964."). The law incorporates the damages caps of 42 U.S.C. § 1981a. Pub. L. No. 117-328, § 104 (a)(3).

[190] Pub. L. No. 117-328, § 104(f).

[191] *Id.* §§ 104 (a)(1), (e)(1), 105(a). The statute calls for rulemaking within one year of enactment. *Id.* § 105(a). The Board of Directors of the Office of Congressional Workplace Rights must promulgate regulations and administer the act for legislative employees. *Id.* § 105(b).

[192] *See* PWF Act, *supra* note 167.

The Family and Medical Leave Act and Unpaid, Job-Protected Leave

The Family and Medical Leave Act (FMLA) requires certain employers to grant unpaid leave for illness and some family responsibilities. Eligible workers may invoke the FMLA to, for example, obtain time off work for pregnancy-related issues, including prenatal care.[193] Most employees may request up to 12 weeks of job-protected leave.

Not all workers are eligible for FMLA leave. Among other requirements, an employee must accrue at least a year of service before taking FMLA leave, and employers of fewer than 50 employees need not offer FMLA leave.[194] Private- and public-sector employees are covered, but members of the armed forces are not.[195] The Department of Labor enforces the FMLA.[196]

The Fair Labor Standards Act and Lactation

The Fair Labor Standards Act of 1938 (FLSA) is probably best known for governing worker pay and hours, but it also requires lactation breaks for nursing mothers.[197] The FLSA affords qualifying employees the right to break time and a private place (not a bathroom) to express breast milk for one year after a child's birth.[198] Employers need not pay workers for break time designated for pumping, but employees who pump during other break times are entitled to compensation on the same terms as employees who use that

---

[193] 29 U.S.C. § 2601; Walter E. Zink II & Jill Gradwohl Schroeder, *Evaluating the Interplay Among FMLA, ADA and Workers' Comp Statutes Isn't Child's Play*, 66 DEF. COUNS. J. 79, 84 (1999). For an overview of the FMLA, see CRS Report R44274, *The Family and Medical Leave Act: An Overview of Title I*, by Sarah A. Donovan (2015).

[194] 29 U.S.C. § 2611(2).

[195] *Id.* §§ 203(e)(2), 2611(4).

[196] *Id.* § 2617(b); *see also* CRS Report R44274, *The Family and Medical Leave Act: An Overview of Title I*, by Sarah A. Donovan (2015).

[197] Fair Labor Standards Act, 29 U.S.C. §§ 207(r), 218c (as amended by the Providing Urgent Maternal Protections (PUMP) for Nursing Mothers Act, Pub. L. No. 117-328, 136 Stat. 4459 (2022)); U.S. DEP'T OF LABOR, WAGES AND THE FAIR LABOR STANDARDS ACT, https://www.dol.gov/agencies/whd/flsa (last visited June 8, 2023); CRS Report R42713, *The Fair Labor Standards Act (FLSA): An Overview*, by Sarah A. Donovan (2023).

[198] 29 U.S.C. §§ 207(r), 218c; PUMP for Nursing Mothers Act, Pub. L. No. 117-328, Div. KK, § 102(a), 136 Stat. 4459 (2022).

break time for other purposes.[199] Separately, existing federal policy calls for all executive branch employers to provide nursing accommodations.[200] Before December 2022, however, those provisions applied only to employees eligible for overtime under the FLSA's Section 7.[201]

In December 2022 Congress expanded FLSA protections for nursing mothers, extending them to previously ineligible workers in the Providing Urgent Maternal Protections (PUMP) for Nursing Mothers Act.[202] Effective immediately, the PUMP for Nursing Mothers Act (passed as part of the Consolidated Appropriations Act of 2023) expands protections to most FLSA-eligible employees.[203] Even as amended, the law does not cover all workers. In particular, employers of fewer than 50 workers need not comply if the requirement would impose an undue hardship.[204]

The PUMP for Nursing Mothers Act also expands available remedies. Potential legal and equitable remedies include hiring, reinstatement, promotion, lost wages, and other damages, including punitive damages.[205]

---

[199] 29 U.S.C. § 207(r)(2), (3); U.S. DEP'T OF LABOR, WAGE & HOUR DIV., FACT SHEET #73: FLSA PROTECTIONS FOR EMPLOYEES TO PUMP BREAST MILK AT WORK (Jan. 2023), https://www.dol.gov/agencies/whd/fact-sheets/73-flsa-break-time-nursing-mothers [hereinafter "FACT SHEET #73"] (last visited June 8, 2023).

[200] JOHN BERRY, OFF. OF PERSONNEL MGMT., MEMORANDUM TO HEADS OF EXEC. DEP'TS & AGENCIES, NURSING MOTHERS IN FEDERAL EMPLOYMENT (Dec. 22, 2010), https://www.dol.gov/sites/dolgov/files/WHD/legacy/files/NMothers FederalEmplymnt.pdf (concluding that, while the 2010 FLSA provisions applied only to overtime-eligible employees, federal agencies should provide reasonable break time for civilian, executive employees).

[201] *Id.*

[202] Enacted as Division KK of the Consolidated Appropriations Act of 2023, the PUMP for Nursing Mothers Act, Pub. L. No. 117-328, Div. KK, 136 Stat. 4459 (2022) moved nursing mother protections from Section 7 of the FLSA and reformulated them as a new Section 18D.

[203] By separating nursing protections from FLSA's Section 7, the new law extended protections to workers not covered under Section 7. These protections now reach FLSA-eligible employees generally, with some enumerated exceptions. Pub. L. No. 117-328, § 102(a); *see also* H.R. REP. NO. 117-102, at 11–12, 21 (2021) (Report from the Committee on Education and Labor) (explaining the effects of moving the provisions in discussing a predecessor bill); U.S. DEP'T OF LABOR, FLSA PROTECTIONS TO PUMP AT WORK, https://www.dol.gov/agencies/whd/pump-at-work (last visited June 8, 2023); FACT SHEET #73, *supra* note 199 (noting the PUMP Act reaches "nearly all FLSA-covered employees").

[204] Pub. L. No. 117-328, § 102(a). The PUMP for Nursing Mothers Act borrows from the ADA's definition of undue hardship, asking courts to consider whether allowing pumping breaks is "causing the employer significant difficulty or expense when considered in relation to the size, financial resources, nature, or structure of the employer's business." *Id.*

[205] *Id.* § 102(b).

These penalties are available for violations after April 28, 2023.[206] The Department of Labor enforces the FLSA.[207]

Executive Order 13152 and Discrimination Based on Parental Status

It addition to the statutory protections described above, federal executive-branch employees— men and women—enjoy protection from intentional discrimination based on parental status.

Executive Order 13152 bars "discrimination in employment because of . . . status as a parent."[208] The Office of Personnel Management (OPM) administers the order, and agencies generally internally investigate and adjudicate complaints.[209] The order does not require accommodations for parents or create pathways to enforcement outside of the agency, such as recourse to EEOC adjudication.[210] While the order does not protect pregnancy per se, it does bar discrimination on account of soon-to-be motherhood.[211] An example of discrimination, OPM has explained, includes stereotypes that parents of young children should not work or lack commitment to work.[212]

---

[206] *Id.* § 103; FACT SHEET #73, *supra* note 199.

[207] U.S. DEP'T OF LABOR, FLSA PROTECTIONS TO PUMP AT WORK https://www.dol.gov/agencies/whd/pump-at-work (last visited June 8, 2023); U.S. DEP'T OF LABOR, COMPLAINTS CAN BE FILED ONLINE, HOW TO FILE A COMPLAINT, https://www.dol.gov/agencies/whd/contact/complaints (last visited June 8, 2023).

[208] Exec. Order No. 13,152, *Further Amendment to Executive Order11,478, Equal Employment Opportunity in Federal Government*, 65 Fed. Reg. 26115 (May 2, 2000). A parent includes a biological parent, adoptive parent, foster parent, step-parent, and others. *Id.*

[209] *Id.*; Complainant v. Dep't of Treasury, EEOC Appeal No. 0120143110, 2015 WL 1635909, at *1 (Mar. 10, 2015) (reflecting agency's internal process).

[210] JANICE R. LACHANCE, OFF. OF PERSONNEL MNGMT., MEMORANDUM FOR HEADS OF DEP'TS & INDEPENDENT ESTABLISHMENTS, GUIDANCE ON ADDRESSING DISCRIMINATION BASED ON STATUS AS A PARENT IN FEDERAL CIVILIAN EMPLOYMENT 2 (Jan. 19, 2001), https://www.nrc.gov/docs/ML0103/ML010310035.pdf.

[211] The order also protects anyone actively seeking custody or adoption of a child. Exec. Order No. 13,152, *Further Amendment to Executive Order 11,478, Equal Employment Opportunity in Federal Government*, 65 Fed. Reg. 26115 (May 2, 2000).

[212] Similar sentiments sometimes play a role in pregnancy discrimination. *See, e.g.*, Int'l Union, United Auto., Aerospace & Agr. Implement Workers of Am., UAW v. Johnson Controls, Inc., 499 U.S. 187, 197–98 (1991); Pacourek v. Inland Steel Co., 858 F. Supp. 1393, 1401 (N.D. Ill. 1994); Jacobson v. Regent Assisted Living, Inc., No. CV-98-564-ST, 1999 WL 373790, at *3 (D. Or. Apr. 9, 1999) (reporting manager asking about employee: "what will her commitment be to the company when she has this baby?").

State Pregnancy Protections

Many states have employment discrimination laws that mirror Title VII, including antidiscrimination measures applicable to pregnancy. In recent years, several states have expanded these laws to include accommodations for pregnant workers.[213] Unlike the PWFA—a separate law providing for pregnancy accommodations—many state laws take the form of amendments to existing laws barring discrimination in employment based on race, sex, religion, and other factors.[214] Sometimes state pregnancy accommodation protections build on those states' disability laws. In Kentucky, for example, pregnancy legislation expanded a requirement of "[r]easonable accommodation[s]," originally intended to benefit workers with disabilities, to include specific job modifications "[f]or an employee's own limitations related to her pregnancy, childbirth, or related medical conditions."[215] Other states have similar measures.[216] Some provisions expressly address pregnant workers' needs for breaks, seating, leave, or other contingencies.[217] Colorado law, for example, states that these may include "more frequent restroom, food, and water breaks; acquisition or modification of equipment or seating; limitations on lifting; temporary transfer to a less strenuous or hazardous position if available, with return to the current position after pregnancy; job restructuring; light duty, if available; assistance with manual labor; or

---

[213] Brianna L. Eaton, Note, Pregnancy Discrimination: Pregnant Women Need More Protection in the Workplace, 64 S.D. L. REV. 244, 262 (2019); Reva B. Siegel, Pregnancy As A Normal Condition of Employment: Comparative and Role-Based Accounts of Discrimination Cutler Lecture, 59 WM. & MARY L. REV. 969, 974 (2018). See, e.g., HAW. CODE R. § 12-46-107 (1990) (implementing Hawaii's Title VII-like antidiscrimination statute and requiring pregnancy accommodations). State regulations, too, may require accommodations.

[214] *See, e.g.*, S.C. CODE ANN. § 1-13-80 (2018); CONN. GEN. STAT. ANN. §§ 46a-60 (2022).

[215] KY. REV. STAT. ANN. § 344.030(6)(b) (2019).

[216] W. VA. CODE ANN. § 5-11B-5 (5) (2014) (stating "'Reasonable accommodation' and 'undue hardship' have the meanings given those terms in section 101 of the Americans with Disabilities Act of 1990"); DEL. CODE ANN. tit. 19, §§ 710-11 (requiring "reasonable accommodations to the known limitations related" to "pregnancy, childbirth, or a related condition, including, but not limited to, lactation").

[217] *See, e.g.*, COLO. REV. STAT. ANN. § 24-34-402.3(4)(b) (2016); NEV. REV. STAT. ANN. § 613.4371 (2017); *see also* W. VA. CODE § 5-11b-4 (2014) (authorizing regulations that "identify some reasonable accommodations addressing known limitations related to pregnancy, childbirth, or related medical conditions").

modified work schedules."[218] State laws also often protect nursing mothers.[219] For some workers, state laws may be more protective than federal laws.

Pregnancy Protections in Context and Potential Reform

While the PDA has for decades barred employers from singling out pregnant workers for adverse action or harassment, critics long called for enhanced protections. Treating pregnant women the same as other workers, accommodations proponents have argued, does not help pregnant workers retain employment.[220] Proposals have generally fallen into two categories: (1) requiring job modifications akin to the "reasonable accommodations" provided for disability, and (2) pregnancy-specific leave entitlements.[221] The PWFA, which parallels the ADA, addressed the first category by focusing on workers' entitlement to pregnancy accommodations.[222] With respect to the second category, advocates for expanded leave and reemployment rights contend that state and federal measures requiring workplace leave to support socially beneficial activities like voting, jury duty, court appearances, and military service may provide paradigms for protecting employment while enabling pregnancy and child care.[223] An overview of these measures can help

---

[218] COLO. REV. STAT. ANN. § 24-34-402.3(4)(b) (2016); *see also* NEV. REV. STAT. ANN. § 613.4371 (2017); VA. CODE ANN. § 2.2-3909 (2021).

[219] NATIONAL CONFERENCE OF STATE LEGISLATURES, BREASTFEEDING STATE LAWS (2021), https://www.ncsl.org/health/breastfeeding-state-laws (last visited June 8, 2023). These include laws requiring pump breaks for employees, see, for example, ARK. CODE ANN. § 11-5-116 (2009); CAL. LAB. CODE § 1030-1033 (2001); D.C. CODE ANN. § 2-1402.82(d)(1) (2007), as well as laws permitting breastfeeding in public. *See, e.g.*, FLA. STAT. ANN. § 383.015 (1993); CAL. CIVIL CODE § 43.3 (1997); 740 ILL. COMP. STAT. ANN. § 137/1 *et. seq.* (2004).

[220] Samuel Issacharoff & Elyse Rosenblum, *Women and the Workplace: Accommodating the Demands of Pregnancy*, 94 COLUM. L. REV. 2154, 2158 (1994); *see also* Siegel, *supra* note 213, at 988.

[221] *See* Areheart, *supra* note 79, at 1128–30; Jeannette Cox, *Pregnancy As "Disability" and the Amended Americans with Disabilities Act*, 53 B.C. L. REV. 443, 449 (2012); Issacharoff & Rosenblum, *supra* note 220 at 2197.

[222] Scholars and advocates had often pointed to the ADA as a starting point or a model for potential legislation. *See supra* note 221. State-law pregnant workers protections often require accommodations, similar to those used for disability. *See supra* notes 215-218. Another potential accommodation analogue is Title VII's religious accommodation provision. Under Title VII's requirements, employers must make changes to workplace rules to accommodate employees' religious practices, unless this poses an "undue hardship on the conduct of the employer's business." 42U.S.C. § 2000e(j).

[223] Bryce Covert, *The American Workplace Still Won't Accommodate Pregnant Workers*, NATION (Aug. 12, 2019), https://www.thenation.com/article/archive/pregnant-workers-

contextualize existing pregnancy protections within employment antidiscrimination law.

Leave entitlements differ from accommodations, as they need not require a showing of disability, known limitation, or reasonableness (as under the ADA or PWFA). As one observer indicated in evaluating FMLA leave entitlements, "treating family and medical leave like leave for jury duty or military service . . . explicitly recognizes the value of caring for others, rather than focusing only on questions of identity and equal treatment."[224] There are a number of statutes that could serve as models for pregnancy-specific leave entitlements. Perhaps the most comprehensive legal regime protecting employment leave is the Uniformed Services Employment and Reemployment Rights Act (USERRA). Through antidiscrimination, antiretaliation, and reemployment provisions, the statute helps military reserve members to complete periodic training and, when needed, extended deployments.[225] One observer characterized USERRA as "possibly the most employee-friendly labor/employment law in effect today."[226] The law's stated purpose is to "eliminat[e] or minimiz[e] the disadvantages to civilian careers and employment which can result from [military] service."[227]

Employers cannot fire, refuse to hire, or refuse to promote a servicemember because of his or her past, present, or future service obligations. Courts borrow from Title VII and similar laws when analyzing causation under USERRA; the Supreme Court has assessed the statute as "very similar to Title VII."[228]

USERRA does more than bar adverse employment actions because of service obligations. The statute protects workers' jobs by requiring that they receive leave without pay during military service. Upon return, a servicemember receives the same status, benefits, and pay at the rate

---

discrimination-workplace-low-wage/ (quoting Gillian Thomas of the American Civil Liberties Union asking employers, "If this were not a pregnancy but if it were jury duty, what would you do?"); Robin R. Runge, *Redefining Leave from Work*, 19 GEO. J. ON POVERTY L. & POL'Y 445, 462 (2012); *see also* CATHERINE R. ALBISTON, INSTITUTIONAL INEQUALITY AND THE MOBILIZATION OF THE FAMILY AND MEDICAL LEAVE ACT: RIGHTS ON LEAVE 73, 135 (2010) (stating that leave-oriented statutes like the FMLA differ from Title VII and the ADA because they do not focus on workers' identities and are "more like legislation that creates job- protected leaves for jury duty or military service than anti-discrimination legislation").

[224] ALBISTON, *supra* note 223, at 135.

[225] 38 U.S.C. § 4311(a).

[226] Kenan Torrans, A Primer on the Uniformed Services Employment and Reemployment Rights Act, 47 MD. B.J. 13 (March 2014).

[227] 38 U.S.C. § 4301(a)(1).

[228] Staub v. Proctor Hosp., 562 U.S. 411, 417 (2011).

previously earned.[229] The servicemember is also entitled to the same promotion opportunities and pay increases available to those who did not take leave for military duties and accrues seniority during deployment.[230] Employers can escape these obligations, however, if their "circumstances have so changed as to make such reemployment impossible or unreasonable."[231]

The FMLA also has protections for military service, allowing a servicemember's next of kin to take 26 weeks of leave to care for the servicemember.[232] On top of federal law's substantial protections, many states provide other benefits to accommodate military service. These benefits include leave rights for military spouses in connection with a deployment.[233]

Aside from military service, legislatures have mandated leave for other endeavors. Federal law and many state laws protect employees who need leave for jury service. Federal law bars employers from discharging employees for federal jury service.[234] Federal employees receive pay for jury service, and federal regulations for unemployment benefits exempt those serving as jurors from requirements that they search for work.[235] Almost all states also bar employers from firing employees because of jury service, and many go further, requiring paid leave for time served as a juror.[236] Other state laws restrict the working hours an employer can require during jury service or bar employers from requiring jurors to use sick leave or vacation to cover their service.[237]

---

[229] 38 U.S.C. § 4313(a); see also Torrans, supra note 226, at 15.

[230] 38 U.S.C. § 4313; see also Molly Weston Williamson, The Meaning of Leave: Understanding Workplace Leave Rights, 22 N.Y.U. J. LEGIS. & PUB. POL'Y 197, 216 (2020) (noting this accrual of seniority during leave is unusual in employment law, "used essentially exclusively in the context of military service").

[231] 38 U.S.C. § 4312(d)(1)(A).

[232] 29 U.S.C. § 2612(3). For covered nonmilitary families, the FMLA affords 12 weeks of leave to care for a family member. *Id.* § 2612(1).

[233] Williamson, *supra* note 230, at 202.

[234] 28 U.S.C. § 1875.

[235] 20 C.F.R. § 615.8(g)(3)(i)(A); OFF. OF PERSONNEL MGMT., FACT SHEET: COURT LEAVE, https://www.opm.gov/policy-data-oversight/pay-leave/leave-administration/fact-sheets/court-leave/ (last visited June 8, 2023).

[236] *See, e.g.*, ALA. CODE § 12-16-8 (1975); CAL. LABOR CODE § 230(a); 705 ILL. COMP. STAT. ANN. § 305/4.1(b) (1991); N.Y. JUD. LAW § 519; Williamson, *supra* note 230, at 201 ("Every state except Montana provides some type of specific workplace protection for those serving jury duty."); Runge, *supra* note 223, at 462; Marianne DelPo Kulow, *Legislating A Family-Friendly Workplace: Should It Be Done in the United States?*, 7 NW. J. L. & SOC. POL'Y 88, 95 (2012). As one analysis concluded, such legislation "reflect[s] the value society places on participating in the justice system." Runge, *supra* note 223 at 462.

[237] Williamson, *supra* note 230, at 209. Some observers describe paid jury duty as a "civic responsibility" employers should shoulder. Jamie Philpotts, *Los Angeles-Based Latham &*

In addition to protections for jury service, bone-marrow or organ donors often receive time off.[238] Some states provide leave for those who volunteer as emergency or disaster service workers.[239] Voting, too, is commonly supported by leave entitlements, mandated in at least 30 states.[240] These types of leave requirements may generally call for shorter leave entitlements than would pregnancy—often a matter of days or even hours rather than weeks or months. They may serve as useful points of comparison, however, because they (unlike many disability accommodations) anticipate a temporary, rather than permanent, alteration of workplace obligations.

Proposed reforms to strengthen protections for pregnant people go beyond workplace leave and accommodation requirements. The Equality Act, passed by the House of Representatives in early 2021, would broaden pregnancy antidiscrimination law beyond employment, applying it in many other areas of public life.[241] The bill includes provisions defining pregnancy discrimination as sex discrimination and further addresses discrimination against breastfeeding women.[242]

Conclusion and Considerations for Congress

A cluster of federal statutes currently protects pregnant workers. As it stands, Title VII, including its PDA provisions, mainly protects pregnant workers from employer bias by barring employers from using pregnancy in employment decisions.[243] The 2022 PWFA mandates pregnancy accommodations at work.[244] The law is modeled on the ADA, which requires accommodations for pregnancy conditions that rise to the level of a disability.[245] How courts and regulators will apply the PWFA, particularly where it departs from established ADA law, remains to be seen. The FMLA provides affirmative benefits for some pregnant workers, most notably unpaid

---

Watkins Was Recently Reprimanded by A Local Federal Judge for Not Allowing a Secretary Paid Leave for Jury Duty, OF COUNSEL, September 21, 1992, at 15 (quoting district judge).

238 Kulow, *supra* note 236, at 95.

239 *Id* at 95–96.

240 *Id.* at 95 n.55.

241 H.R. 5, 117th Cong. §§ 3, 4, 6, 9 (2021); *see also* S. 393, 117th Cong. § 2 (2021).

242 H.R. 5, 117th Cong. §§ 2, 9; *see also* S. 393 §§ 2, 9.

243 *See supra* notes 4–27 and accompanying text.

244 Pregnant Workers Fairness Act, Pub. L. No. 117-328, 136 Stat. 4459 (2022).

245 *See supra* notes 141–163 and accompanying text.

leave for eligible employees.[246] The FLSA, as amended by the PUMP for Nursing Mothers Act, separately requires break time and other benefits for nursing mothers.[247]

Over the years, Congress has expanded pregnant workers' protections. Congress clarified Title VII's application to pregnancy with the PDA; broadened the definition of disability within the ADA to include temporary disabilities, enhancing protection for pregnant employees (among others); and passed the PWFA and PUMP for Nursing Mothers Act.[248] Several states have also passed pregnancy accommodations laws to supplement existing antidiscrimination measures.[249]

Courts have helped shape pregnancy protections as well. The Supreme Court's decision in *Gilbert* motivated passage of the PDA.[250] More recently, the Court's application of Title VII's PDA provisions in *Young* raised questions as to whether and when pregnancy accommodations are required under that law.[251] Congress then passed a separate law, the PWFA, mandating pregnancy accommodations. The result is expansive yet piecemeal legislation regarding the treatment of pregnancy in the workplace.

If Congress seeks to enhance, restrict, or consolidate these measures, it may choose to amend Title VII, the PWFA, the ADA, the FLSA, or the FMLA. Congress may wish to take note of what issues emerge in courts' and regulators' application of the PWFA, for instance. With respect to that law, Congress might consider enumerating, as some state laws do, presumptively reasonable pregnancy accommodations.[252] It could also exclude specific accommodations.

In considering new measures, federal and state legislation in contexts unrelated to disabilities or discrimination may provide models for enacting pregnancy-specific job protection and leave options. Congress might consider enacting pregnancy-specific leave entitlements beyond those qualifying as reasonable accommodations under the PWFA, making leave available without

---

[246] *See supra* notes 193–195 and accompanying text.

[247] *See supra* notes 197–207 and accompanying text.

[248] 42 U.S.C. § 2000e(k); *id.* § 12102(4)(A); ADA Amendments Act of 2008, Pub. L. No. 110-325, 122 Stat. 3553; Pregnant Workers Fairness Act, Pub. L. No. 117-328, 136 Stat. 4459 (2022); PUMP for Nursing Mothers Act, Pub. L. No. 117-328, Div. KK, § 102(a), 136 Stat. 4459 (2022); Young v. United Parcel Serv., Inc., 575 U.S. 206, 252 (2015) (Kennedy, J., dissenting); *supra* notes 16–20 and 165–192 and accompanying text.

[249] *See supra* notes 213–216 and accompanying text.

[250] 42 U.S.C. § 2000e(k); *supra* notes 15–20.

[251] *See supra* notes 78–130 and accompanying text.

[252] *See, e.g.*, COLO. REV. STAT. ANN. § 24-34-402.3(4)(b) (2016); NEV. REV. STAT. ANN. § 613.4371(2017); VA. CODE ANN. § 2.2-3909 (2021).

requiring a pregnancy-related impairment, reasonableness, or lack of undue hardship. For example, Congress could expand FMLA leave for pregnant workers currently ineligible because of employer size or length of employment. Congress could also offer FMLA leave specific to pregnancy and childbearing (the FMLA, for example, offers additional leave for caring for a servicemember).

Chapter 9

Equal Employment Opportunity Commission: Implementation of the Pregnant Workers Fairness Act*

U.S. Government Accountability Office

The Honorable Bernard Sanders Chairman
The Honorable Bill Cassidy Ranking Member
Committee on Health, Education, Labor, and Pensions
United States Senate

The Honorable Virginia Foxx Chairwoman
The Honorable Bobby Scott Ranking Member
Committee on Education and the Workforce
House of Representatives

Pursuant to section 801(a)(2)(A) of title 5, United States Code, this is our report on a major rule promulgated by the Equal Employment Opportunity Commission (EEOC) entitled "Implementation of the Pregnant Workers Fairness Act" (RIN: 3046-AB30). We received the rule on April 15, 2024. It was published in the Federal Register as a final rule and interpretive guidance on April 19, 2024. 89 Fed. Reg. 29096. The effective date is June 18, 2024.

According to EEOC, the final rule implements the Pregnant Workers Fairness Act, included as part of the Consolidated Appropriations Act, 2023, Pub. L. No. 117-328, div. II, 136 Stat. 4459, 6084 (2022), and codified at 42

---

* This is an edited, reformatted and augmented version of the United States Government Accountability Office Publication No. B-336251, dated May 1, 2024.

In: Navigating Pregnancy Challenges
Editor: Javier Giles
ISBN: 979-8-89530-857-8

U.S.C. §§ 2000gg–2000gg-6. EEOC states that this Act requires a covered entity to provide reasonable accommodations to a qualified employee's or applicant's known limitations related to, affected by, or arising out of pregnancy, childbirth, or related medical conditions, unless the accommodation will cause an undue hardship on the operation of the business of the covered entity.

Enclosed is our assessment of EEOC's compliance with the procedural steps required by section 801(a)(1)(B)(i) through (iv) of title 5 with respect to the rule. If you have any questions about this report or wish to contact GAO officials responsible for the evaluation work relating to the subject matter of the rule, please contact Charlie McKiver, Assistant General Counsel, at (202) 512-5992.

Shirley A. Jones
Managing Associate General Counsel

Enclosure
cc: Carol R. Miaskoff Legal Counsel
Equal Employment Opportunity Commission

Report Under 5 U.S.C. § 801(A)(2)(A) on a Major Rule Issued by the Equal Employment Opportunity Commission Entitled "Implementation of the Pregnant Workers Fairness Act" (Rin: 3046-Ab30)

(i) Cost-benefit analysis

The Equal Employment Opportunity Commission (EEOC) prepared a Final Regulatory Impact Analysis. EEOC estimated the cost of the rule to be between $466.71 million and $484.71 million in the first year, and between $14.82 million and $32.82 million annually thereafter. EEOC identified the two main expected costs associated with the rule as: (1) annual costs associated with providing reasonable accommodations to qualified applicants and employees with known limitations related to, affected by, or arising out of pregnancy, childbirth, or related medical conditions by employers in states that do not currently have such a requirement; and (2) one-time administrative costs for covered entities, which include becoming familiar with the rule, posting new equal employment opportunity (EEO) posters, and updating EEO policies and handbooks.

EEOC stated that the non-quantifiable benefits of the rule include: improved maternal and infant health; improved economic security for pregnant employees; increased equity, human dignity, and fairness; improved clarity of enforcement standards and efficiencies in litigation; and decreased costs related to employee turnover for covered entities. EEOC stated that while those benefits cannot be fully quantified and monetized, the agency concluded that, consistent with Executive Order No. 13563, the benefits will justify the costs.

(ii) Agency actions relevant to the Regulatory Flexibility Act (RFA), 5 U.S.C. §§ 603–605, 607, and 609

The Chair of EEOC certified that this final rule will not have a significant economic impact on a substantial number of small entities. Although EEOC determined that the rule will impact a substantial number of small entities, EEOC determined that the economic impact on entities affected will not be significant.

(iii) Agency actions relevant to sections 202–205 of the Unfunded Mandates Reform Act of 1995, 2 U.S.C. §§ 1532–1535

EEOC determined that the Unfunded Mandates Reform Act of 1995 (UMRA) does not apply to the Pregnant Workers Fairness Act due to a provision (2 U.S.C. § 1503) that excludes from UMRA's coverage any provision in a final regulation that, among other things, enforces constitutional rights of individuals or establishes or enforces any statutory rights that prohibit discrimination on the basis of race, color, religion, sex, national origin, age, handicap, or disability.

(iv) Agency actions relevant to the Administrative Pay-As-You-Go-Act of 2023, Pub. L. No. 118-5, div. B, title III, 137 Stat 31 (June 3, 2023)

Section 270 of the Administrative Pay-As-You-Go-Act of 2023 amended 5 U.S.C. § 801(a)(2)(A) to require GAO to assess agency compliance with the Act, which establishes requirements for administrative actions that affect direct spending, in GAO's major rule reports. In guidance to Executive Branch agencies, issued on September 1, 2023, the Office of Management and Budget (OMB) instructed that agencies should include a statement explaining that either: "the Act does not apply to this rule because it does not increase direct spending; the Act does not apply to this rule because it meets one of the Act's exemptions (and specifying the relevant exemption); the OMB Director granted a waiver of the Act's requirements pursuant to section 265(a)(1) or (2) of the Act; or the agency has submitted a notice or written opinion to the OMB Director as required by section 263(a) or (b) of the Act" in their submissions of rules to GAO under the Congressional Review Act. OMB, Memorandum for the Heads of Executive Departments and Agencies, Subject: Guidance for Implementation of the Administrative Pay-As-You-Go Act of 2023, M-23-21 (Sept. 1, 2023), at 11–12. OMB also states that directives in the memorandum that supplement the requirements in the Act do not apply to proposed rules that have already been submitted to the Office of Information and Regulatory Affairs, however agencies must comply with any applicable requirements of the Act before finalizing such rules.

EEOC did not discuss the Act in the rule or in its submission to us.

(v) Other relevant information or requirements under acts and executive orders Administrative Procedure Act, 5 U.S.C. §§ 551 et seq.

On August 11, 2023, EEOC issued a proposed rule. 88 Fed. Reg. 54714. EEOC received 98,600 comments, several of which were signed by multiple individuals. EEOC stated that the vast majority of the comments were form comments that were identical or slightly altered versions of a few base form comments. EEOC responded to comments in this final rule.

Paperwork Reduction Act (PRA), 44 U.S.C. §§ 3501–3520

EEOC determined that there is no new requirement for information collection associated with this final rule.

Statutory authorization for the rule

EEOC promulgated this final rule pursuant to sections 2000gg et seq. of title 42, United States Code.

Executive Order No. 12866 (Regulatory Planning and Review)

EEOC determined that this final rule is significant under the Order and submitted it to OMB for review.

Executive Order No. 13132 (Federalism)

EEOC determined that this final rule does not have federalism implications. EEOC stated that the rule does not limit or expand the relevant statutory definitions describing the application of the Pregnant Workers Fairness Act to states, and the rule will not have substantial direct effects on the relationship between the national government and the states, or on the distribution of power and responsibilities among the various levels of government.

Chapter 10

New Federal Protections for Pregnant and Nursing Workers*

April J. Anderson

Several federal laws protect workers during nursing and pregnancy, but two new federal laws, passed as part of the Consolidated Appropriations Act of 2023, go into effect this year and expand those protections in certain ways. The Providing Urgent Maternal Protections for Nursing Mothers Act (PUMP for Nursing Mothers Act), Pub. L. No. 117- 328, 136 Stat. 4459 (2022), expands protections for nursing mothers, requiring break time and appropriate facilities for workers to express breast milk. The Pregnant Workers Fairness Act (PWFA), Pub. L. No. 117-328, 136 Stat. 4459 (2022), requires employers to modify workplace rules and conditions where needed to accommodate pregnancy- related limitations, provided that an accommodation is reasonable and does not present an undue hardship to the employer.

This In Focus summarizes these two statutes, placing them in context and highlighting the ways they draw on and differ from existing laws. It explains who qualifies for accommodations, what employers must provide, and the limits of employers' responsibilities.

---

* This is an edited, reformatted and augmented version of Congressional Research Service Publication No. IF12392, dated April 28, 2023.

In: Navigating Pregnancy Challenges
Editor: Javier Giles
ISBN: 979-8-89530-857-8

Providing Urgent Maternal Protections for Nursing Mothers Act (PUMP for Nursing Mothers Act)

In the PUMP for Nursing Mothers Act, Congress expanded existing protections for nursing mothers. The Fair Labor Standards Act of 1938 (FLSA), 29 U.S.C. §§ 201 et seq., requires lactation breaks for some nursing mothers. The PUMP for Nursing Mothers Act takes those protections, which previously covered certain overtime-eligible employees, and applies them to nearly all FLSA-covered workers. The new law's substantive requirements largely track the earlier FLSA provisions. They afford qualifying employees break time and a private place (not a bathroom) to express breast milk. The protections apply for one year after a child's birth. Employers need not pay workers for break time designated for pumping, but employees who pump during break times are entitled to compensation on the same terms as those who use their break times for other purposes. The law's enhanced coverage takes effect immediately.

Even as amended, the law does not cover certain workers. In particular, employers with fewer than 50 workers need not comply if doing so would impose an undue hardship. An "undue hardship" is defined in similar terms as Title I of the Americans with Disabilities Act (ADA), 42 U.S.C. §§ 12111–12117, governing workplace disability accommodations: "causing the employer significant difficulty or expense when considered in relation to the size, financial resources, nature, or structure of the employer's business."

The amendments also expand available remedies. Potential legal and equitable remedies include hiring, reinstatement, promotion, lost wages, and other damages, including punitive damages. These penalties are available for violations after April 28, 2023. The Department of Labor enforces the FLSA, including accepting worker complaints. The act does not address congressional employment or amend the Congressional Accountability Act of 1995 (CAA), which specifies FLSA provisions applicable to legislative employees.

The Pregnant Workers Fairness Act (PWFA)

The PWFA requires reasonable accommodations for worker limitations arising from "pregnancy, childbirth, or related medical conditions." The PWFA does not define this phrase, but the same phrase is also used in Title

VII of the Civil Rights Act of 1964 (Title VII), 42 U.S.C. §§ 2000e et seq. (barring discrimination in employment). Courts construing Title VII have held it to cover complications during pregnancy, such as nausea and lifting restrictions; recovery from childbirth including by caesarian section; and postpartum conditions such as depression. Although there is some judicial variation, some courts have concluded that "related medical conditions" can also include fertility treatment, lactation, and abortion.

The PWFA provides that its requirement for "reasonable accommodations" has the same meaning as in the ADA. Under the ADA, courts have held that a reasonable accommodation is a modification of workplace rules or practices that is feasible or plausible in most cases.

Reasonable accommodations for pregnancy might include seating, access to drinking water, bathroom breaks, and light duty. Whether a specific accommodation is required hinges on the facts of each case; reasonableness depends on the employee's limitations and the workplace circumstances.

Under the PWFA's terms, and in line with its ADA model, an employer need not provide an accommodation that imposes an "undue hardship" on business operations. This also requires a case-by-case analysis, considering such factors as the nature and cost of the accommodation, the employer's resources, and the size and function of its workforce. The employer bears the burden of showing an undue hardship once the worker identifies a reasonable accommodation. As with the ADA, the PWFA obliges employers and employees to negotiate in good faith to determine appropriate accommodations. ADA case law has not produced bright-line rules governing the fact-specific, individualized assessment of what constitutes a reasonable accommodation or an undue burden.

Like the ADA and many other antidiscrimination measures, the PWFA bars retaliation against a worker who has requested an accommodation, has opposed any practice barred by the PWFA, or has helped someone make a complaint.

The PWFA, however, differs from the ADA in notable ways. While the ADA requires that disabled employees be able to perform the essential functions of their job, the PWFA would protect employees who cannot perform an essential function if they can resume it in the "near future" and can be reasonably accommodated. The PWFA also directly addresses the potential concern of mandatory leave, requiring that employers not force a qualified employee to take leave if another accommodation would allow the worker to remain on the job. The law states, however, that it will not require modification of any employer-sponsored health plan to "pay for or cover any particular item, procedure, or treatment."

The PWFA also covers more workers than the ADA, as it includes those who do not claim an impairment within the ADA's definition of a "disability." The statute requires accommodations for a pregnancy-related "known limitation," which is a "physical or mental condition related to, affected by, or arising out of pregnancy, childbirth, or related medical conditions . . . whether or not such condition meets the definition of disability." While there is a substantial body of precedent applying the ADA's standard defining "disability," the scope of this new, "known limitation" standard may require further judicial elaboration. The new category, "known limitation," stands in contrast to many other PWFA provisions. In other areas, as in defining "undue hardship" and "reasonable accommodation," the PWFA follows prior statutes rather than introducing new rules.

Regarding its scope of coverage, the PWFA, like the ADA and Title VII, applies to employers of 15 or more workers. It protects job applicants, federal workers, and state workers (with sovereign immunity for state employers being waived). Legislative employees, too, are covered through a cross-reference to the CAA. The PWFA applies to religious employers, but it incorporates Title VII's exemption allowing religious entities to require workers to adhere to the entity's own faith and religious principles.

Enforcement procedures and remedies in the new law track those of Title VII. The PWFA grants the Equal Employment Opportunity Commission (EEOC) and the Attorney General enforcement authority and charges the EEOC with issuing regulations, including providing examples of reasonable accommodations. The Board of Directors of the Office of Congressional Workplace Rights must promulgate regulations and administer the act for federal legislative employees. Remedies can include equitable relief, compensatory damages, punitive damages, and attorneys' fees. The law goes into effect on June 27, 2023.

Other Protections for Pregnant Workers

Other protections still apply to pregnant workers. The Pregnancy Discrimination Act (PDA), in Title VII, protects job applicants and employees from adverse action because of pregnancy or related conditions. The law also addresses harassment based on pregnancy. As construed by the Supreme Court in Young v. United Parcel Service, 575 U.S. 206 (2015), the PDA does not generally require employers to accommodate pregnant workers; this limitation appears to have motivated some PWFA proponents in passing the new law. A worker would rely on Title VII, however, for claims of pregnancy-related adverse action aside from a refusal to provide accommodations.

Other statutes also support pregnant workers. Many workers can invoke the Family and Medical Leave Act (FMLA) for unpaid leave related to childbearing. Some pregnant people face pregnancy-related impairments serious enough to satisfy the ADA's definition of a "disability," and many workers may, along with any PWFA claims, bring ADA claims for accommodations. See CRS In Focus IF12227, The Americans with Disabilities Act: A Brief Overview, by Abigail A. Graber. The Rehabilitation Act of 1973 creates similar protections for workers in federally funded programs and most federal agencies. In addition, many states have enacted laws protecting pregnant workers in recent years, including requirements for pregnancy accommodations and nursing breaks. The PWFA does not preempt more protective state laws.

Considerations for Congress

Over the years, Congress has expanded pregnant workers' protections through piecemeal legislation. Congress may choose to make no further changes. Should it seek to enhance or consolidate protections further, Congress may choose to amend Title VII, the PWFA, the ADA, or the FMLA. Congress might consider enumerating, as some state laws do, presumptively reasonable pregnancy accommodations.

Alternatively, while the PWFA addresses accommodations, Congress might consider enacting pregnancy-specific leave entitlements beyond those qualifying as reasonable accommodations under the PWFA. Congress could make leave available without requiring a pregnancy-related impairment, reasonableness, or lack of undue hardship. For example, Congress could expand the FMLA leave for pregnant workers currently ineligible because of employer size or length of employment. It could also offer FMLA leave specific to pregnancy and childbearing (the FMLA, for example, offers additional leave for caring for a servicemember). Other statutes include leave, promotions, and reemployment for those who leave work for such activities as jury duty or military service.

In any measures defining pregnancy protections, Congress may delineate coverage, deciding whether to exclude smaller employers or religious employers. Congress could consider provisions specific to federal workers, such as amending the CAA to include the PUMP for Nursing Mothers Act among FLSA protections for legislative employees.

Chapter 11

Supporting Pregnant and Parenting Women and Families Act*

Committee on Ways and Means

I. Summary and Background

A. Purpose and Summary

H.R. 6918, as amended, the ''Supporting Pregnant and Parenting Women and Families Act,'' as ordered reported by the Committee on Ways and Means on January 11, 2024 prohibits the Department of Health of Human Services from finalizing, implementing, or enforcing the Notice of Proposed Rulemaking titled, ''Strengthening Temporary Assistance for Needy Families (TANF) as a Safety Net and Work Program,'' proposed at 88 FR 67697, or any substantially similar regulation, as it applies to expenditures for pregnancy centers. Introduced by Rep. Michelle Fischbach (R–MN), Rep. Claudia Tenney (R–NY), and Rep. Chris Smith (R–NJ), this bill protects state flexibility to provide federal TANF funds to pregnancy centers that support protecting the life of the mother and unborn child that offer resources and services including counseling, prenatal and pregnancy education, pregnancy testing, diapers, baby clothes, or other material supports.

* This is an edited, reformatted and augmented version of the Report of the Committee on Ways and Means, committed to the Committee of the Whole House on the State of the Union and ordered to be printed, Publication No. 118–349, dated January 16, 2024.

In: Navigating Pregnancy Challenges
Editor: Javier Giles
ISBN: 979-8-89530-857-8

B. Background and Need for Legislation

Temporary Assistance for Needy Families (TANF) is a key federal program in the fight against poverty. TANF provides $16.5 billion in federal funding to states to further four statutory purposes:[1]

- Provide assistance to needy families so that children can be cared for in their own home or in the home of relatives;
- End the dependence of needy parents on government benefits by promoting job preparation, work, and marriage;
- Prevent and reduce incidence out-of-wedlock pregnancies; and
- Encourage the formation of two-parent families.

On October 2, 2023, the Department of Health and Human Services (HHS) issued a Notice of Proposed Rulemaking (NPRM), ''Strengthening Temporary Assistance for Needy Families (TANF) as a Safety Net and Work Program'' that includes several regulatory reforms to TANF, as well as several technical and administrative changes.[2] One of the proposed regulatory changes in this rule is to clarify when an expenditure is ''reasonably calculated to accomplish a TANF purpose'' to increase the thresholds for states to prove their non-assistance spending meets one of TANF's statutory purposes. This proposed change to TANF regulations are at Subpart B, Section 263.11, which pertain to uses of federal TANF funds that are considered to be improper. The proposed rule would amend this section of the regulations by adding a new subpart (c) to clarify that if an expenditure does not appear to HHS to be reasonably calculated to accomplish a purpose of TANF, a state must show that a ''reasonable person'' would consider the use of funds to be within one or more of the four statutory purposes.

In their explanation of this proposed change, HHS singles out pregnancy centers and preemptively suggests state spending on these organizations would no longer be an allowable TANF expenditure. In the preamble of the proposed rule, HHS states:

> ''[P]rograms that only or primarily provide pregnancy counseling to women only after they become pregnant likely do not meet the reasonable person standard because the connection to preventing and

[1] 42 U.S.C. 601.

[2] RIN 0970–AC99.

reducing out-of-wedlock pregnancies is tenuous or non-existent, and therefore do not accomplish purpose three.''[3]

Pregnancy centers are non-profit organizations that have a pro-life mission and provide services to pregnant women and families including pregnancy testing, testing for sexually transmitted diseases, prenatal and pregnancy education, ultrasounds, adoption referrals, diapers, baby clothes, linkages to housing, and other material supports. Over 2,700 pregnancy centers across the country aided nearly two million people in 2019.[4] Services and material assistance provided by pregnancy centers had an estimated value of over $358 million annually. At least five states in 2023 distributed a portion of their TANF funding to pregnancy centers, including Indiana, Louisiana, Missouri, Ohio, and Pennsylvania.[5]

HHS's proposed rule inaccurately describes pregnancy centers as limited to ''only or primarily provid[ing] pregnancy counseling to women only after they become pregnant'' and only relevant for the ''prevent and reduce incidence out-of-wedlock pregnancies'' and TANF purpose.[6] However, pregnancy centers clearly meet other TANF purposes; for example, by providing material support and assistance to women in need so children can be cared for in their own home and by reducing dependence on government assistance. Documented pregnancy centers services include parenting classes, training in life skills, sexual risk avoidance education, promoting responsible paternity, promoting marriage, care coordination, housing and support services through maternity homes, assistance with job searching, reducing dependence on government and much more.[7]

Furthermore, the changes in the proposed rule are in clear violation of Congressional restrictions placed on the Department's ability to regulate. When TANF was created with bipartisan support and signed into law by President Clinton in 1996, the overarching goal and stated purpose in statute

---

[3] 88 FR 67705.

[4] Charlotte Lozier Institute, ''A Legacy of Life and Love: Pregnancy Centers Stand the Test of Time'', October 21, 2020, https://lozierinstitute.org/wp-content/uploads/2023/01/Pregnancy-Center-Report-2020_FINAL.pdf.

[5] Jeanneane Maxon, Charlotte Lozier Institute, ''Fact Sheet: State Alternatives to Abortion Funding'', June 28, 2022, updated on October 13, 2023, https://lozier institute.org/fact-sheet-state-alternatives-to-abortion-funding/.

[6] 88 FR 67705.

[7] Amanda Stirone Mansfield, Charlotte Lozier Institute, ''Alternatives to Abortion Programs: Support for Mothers and Families,'' February 14, 2022, https://lozierinstitute.org/alternatives-to-abortion-programs-support-for-mothers-and-families.

was ''to increase the flexibility of States.''[8] Likewise, the Committee report emphasized the importance of state flexibility seven times and stated that TANF's purpose is ''to increase state flexibility in providing assistance to needy families . . .''[9] To protect this purpose, Congress explicitly limited the ability of the Executive branch from issuing regulations for the TANF program:

> Sec. 417 Limitations on Federal Authority.[10] No officer or employee of the Federal Government may regulate the conduct of States under this part of enforce any provision of this part, except to the extent expressly provided in this part.

Pregnancy centers are an important alternative for expectant mothers. This bill protects state flexibility to provide federal TANF funds to pregnancy centers that support protecting the life of the mother and unborn child that offer resources and services including but not limited to relationship counseling, prenatal and pregnancy education, pregnancy testing, diapers, baby clothes, or other material supports.

C. Legislative History

Background

H.R. 6918 was introduced on January 9, 2024, and was referred to the Committee on Ways and Means.

Committee Hearings

The Committee has held the following hearing:

On July 12, 2023, the Committee on Ways and Means Subcommittee on Work and Welfare held a hearing titled, ''Where is all the Welfare Money Going? Reclaiming TANF Non-Assistance Dollars to Lift Americans Out of Poverty,'' to hear from state officials and administrators about needed reforms to balance accountability and state flexibility in TANF non-assistance spending.

---

[8] 42 U.S.C. 601.
[9] H.R. Conference Report No 104–15 (1996).
[10] 42 U.S.C. 617.

Committee Action

The Committee on Ways and Means marked up H.R. 6918, the ''Supporting Pregnant and Parenting Women and Families Act'', on January 11, 2023, and ordered the bill, as amended, favorably reported (with a quorum being present).

D. Designated Hearing

Pursuant to clause 3(c)(6) of rule XIII, the following hearing was used to develop and consider: ''Where is all the Welfare Money Going? Reclaiming TANF Non-Assistance Dollars to Lift Americans Out of Poverty'' hearing held on July 12, 2023.

II. Explanation of the Bill

Reasons for Change

Section 1. The Committee believes the title accurately reflects the content of the bill.

Section 2. The Committee believes that preventing the Department of Health and Human Services from finalizing, implementing, or enforcing the Notice of Proposed Rulemaking titled, ''Strengthening Temporary Assistance for Needy Families (TANF) as a Safety Net and Work Program,'' proposed at 88 FR 67697, or any substantially similar regulation, as it applies to expenditures for pregnancy centers is cost-effective, protects state flexibility on the use of federal TANF funds in accordance with Part A Title IV of the Social Security Act, and will benefit the pregnant and parenting women and families served by pregnancy centers.

Explanation of Provisions

Section 1. This section provides the short title, the Supporting Pregnant and Parenting Women and Families Act.

Section 2. This section prohibits the Department of Health of Human Services from finalizing, implementing, or enforcing the Notice of Proposed

Rulemaking titled, ''Strengthening Temporary Assistance for Needy Families (TANF) as a Safety Net and Work Program,'' proposed at 88 FR 67697, or any substantially similar regulation, as it applies to expenditures for pregnancy centers. This section defines ''pregnancy centers'' to mean organizations that support protecting the life of the mother and unborn child that offer resources and services including but not limited to relationship counseling, prenatal and pregnancy education, pregnancy testing, diapers, baby clothes, or other material supports.

Effective Date

The bill would become effective upon enactment.

III. Votes of the Committee

In compliance with the Rules of the House of Representatives, the following statement is made concerning the vote of the Committee on Ways and Means during the markup consideration of H.R. 6918, the ''Supporting Pregnant and Parenting Women and Families Act'' on January 11, 2024.

The vote on the amendment offered by Ms. DelBene to the amendment in the nature of a substitute to H.R. 6918, which would prohibit the legislation from going into effect unless the Secretary of Health and Human Services finds implementation would not result in funds being made available to any organization that presents itself as providing unbiased reproductive health information or counseling, but that covertly intends to discourage pregnant individuals from seeking or accessing abortion services was not agreed to by a roll call vote of 17 yeas to 23 nays (with a quorum being present). The vote was as follows:

Representative	Yea	Nay	Present	Representative	Yea	Nay	Present
Mr. Smith (MO)		X		Mr. Neal	X		
Mr. Buchanan		X		Mr. Doggett	X		
Mr. Smith (NE)		X		Mr. Thompson	X		
Mr. Kelly		X		Mr. Larson	X		
Mr. Schweikert		X		Mr. Blumenauer	X		
Mr. LaHood		X		Mr. Pascrell	X		
Dr. Wenstrup		X		Mr. Davis	X		
Mr. Arrington		X		Ms. Sa´nchez	X		

Representative	Yea	Nay	Present	Representative	Yea	Nay	Present
Dr. Ferguson		X		Mr. Higgins	X		
Mr. Estes		X		Ms. Sewell			
Mr. Smucker		X		Ms. DelBene	X		
Mr. Hern		X		Ms. Chu	X		
Ms. Miller		X		Ms. Moore	X		
Dr. Murphy		X		Mr. Kildee	X		
Mr. Kustoff		X		Mr. Beyer	X		
Mr. Fitzpatrick				Mr. Evans	X		
Mr. Steube				Mr. Schneider	X		
Ms. Tenney		X		Mr. Panetta	X		
Mrs. Fischbach		X					
Mr. Moore		X					
Mrs. Steel		X					
Ms. Van Duyne		X					
Mr. Feenstra		X					
Ms. Malliotakis		X					
Mr. Carey		X					

In compliance with the Rules of the House of Representatives, the following statement is made concerning the vote of the Committee on Ways and Means during the markup consideration of H.R. 6918, the ''Supporting Pregnant and Parenting Women and Families Act'' on January 11, 2024.

The vote on the amendment offered by Ms. Chu to the amendment in the nature of a substitute to H.R. 6918, which would prohibit the legislation from going into effect unless the Secretary of Health and Human Services determines that there will be no negative medical or economic effects on women seeking abortion care who are directed to crisis pregnancy centers was not agreed to by a roll call vote of 17 yeas to 22 nays (with a quorum being present). The vote was as follows:

Representative	Yea	Nay	Present	Representative	Yea	Nay	Present
Mr. Smith (MO)		X		Mr. Neal	X		
Mr. Buchanan		X		Mr. Doggett	X		
Mr. Smith (NE)		X		Mr. Thompson	X		
Mr. Kelly ..		X		Mr. Larson	X		
Mr. Schweikert		X		Mr. Blumenauer	X		
Mr. LaHood		X		Mr. Pascrell	X		
Dr. Wenstrup		X		Mr. Davis	X		
Mr. Arrington		X		Ms. Sa´nchez	X		
Dr. Ferguson		X		Mr. Higgins	X		
Mr. Estes		X		Ms. Sewell			
Mr. Smucker		X		Ms. DelBene	X		
Mr. Hern		X		Ms. Chu	X		
Ms. Miller		X		Ms. Moore	X		

Representative	Yea	Nay	Present	Representative	Yea	Nay	Present
Dr. Murphy				Mr. Kildee	X		
Mr. Kustoff		X		Mr. Beyer	X		
Mr. Fitzpatrick				Mr. Evans	X		
Mr. Steube				Mr. Schneider.	X		
Ms. Tenney		X		Mr. Panetta	X		
		X					
Mr. Moore		X					
Mrs. Steel		X					
Ms. Van Duyne		X					
Mr. Feenstra.		X					
Ms. Malliotakis		X					
Mr. Carey		X					

In compliance with the Rules of the House of Representatives, the following statement is made concerning the vote of the Committee on Ways and Means during the markup consideration of H.R. 6918, the ''Supporting Pregnant and Parenting Women and Families Act'' on January 11, 2024.

The vote on the amendment offered by Ms. Sanchez to the amendment in the nature of a substitute to H.R. 6918, which would prohibit the legislation from going into effect unless the Secretary of Health and Human Services certifies that no Temporary Assistance to Needy Families funds or resources are used to make coercive referrals to Crisis Pregnancy Centers that provide misleading or deceptive information was not agreed to by a roll call vote of 18 yeas to 22 nays (with a quorum being present). The vote was as follows:

Representative	Yea	Nay	Present	Representative	Yea	Nay	Present
Mr. Smith (MO)		X		Mr. Neal	X		
Mr. Buchanan		X		Mr. Doggett	X		
Mr. Smith (NE)		X		Mr. Thompson	X		
Mr. Kelly		X		Mr. Larson	X		
Mr. Schweikert		X		Mr. Blumenauer	X		
Mr. LaHood		X		Mr. Pascrell	X		
Dr. Wenstrup		X		Mr. Davis	X		
Mr. Arrington		X		Ms. Sa´nchez	X		
Dr. Ferguson		X		Mr. Higgins	X		
Mr. Estes		X		Ms. Sewell	X		
Mr. Smucker		X		Ms. DelBene	X		
Mr. Hern		X		Ms. Chu	X		
Ms. Miller		X		Ms. Moore	X		
Dr. Murphy				Mr. Kildee	X		
Mr. Kustoff		X	..	Mr. Beyer	X		
Mr. Fitzpatrick				Mr. Evans	X		
Mr. Steube				Mr. Schneider	X		
Ms. Tenney		X		Mr. Panetta	X		

Representative	Yea	Nay	Present	Representative	Yea	Nay	Present
Mrs. Fischbach		X					
Mr. Moore		X					
Mrs. Steel		X					
Ms. Van Duyne		X					
Mr. Feenstra		X					
Ms. Malliotakis		X					
Mr. Carey		X					

In compliance with the Rules of the House of Representatives, the following statement is made concerning the vote of the Committee on Ways and Means during the markup consideration of H.R. 6918, the ''Supporting Pregnant and Parenting Women and Families Act'' on January 11, 2024.

The vote on the amendment offered by Ms. Moore to the amendment in the nature of a substitute to H.R. 6918, which would prohibit the legislation from going into effect unless the Secretary of Health and Human Services determines that all families in the United States with a child under 5 years of age, where the family has a gross annual income that is less than the poverty line, have guaranteed access to income support, housing, and child care was not agreed to by a roll call vote of 18 yeas to 23 nays (with a quorum being present). The vote was as follows:

Representative	Yea	Nay	Present	Representative	Yea	Nay	Present
Mr. Smith (MO)		X		Mr. Neal	X		
Mr. Buchanan		X		Mr. Doggett	X		
Mr. Smith (NE)		X		Mr. Thompson	X		
Mr. Kelly		X		Mr. Larson	X		
Mr. Schweikert		X		Mr. Blumenauer	X		
Mr. LaHood		X		Mr. Pascrell	X		
Dr. Wenstrup		X		Mr. Davis	X		
Mr. Arrington		X		Ms. Sa´nchez	X		
Dr. Ferguson		X		Mr. Higgins	X		
Mr. Estes		X		Ms. Sewell	X		
Mr. Smucker		X		Ms. DelBene	X		
Mr. Hern		X		Ms. Chu	X		
Ms. Miller		X		Ms. Moore	X		
Dr. Murphy		X		Mr. Kildee	X		
Mr. Kustoff		X		Mr. Beyer	X		
Mr. Fitzpatrick				Mr. Evans	X		
Mr. Steube				Mr. Schneider	X		
Ms. Tenney		X		Mr. Panetta	X		
Mrs. Fischbach		X					
Mr. Moore		X					
Mrs. Steel		X					
Ms. Van Duyne		X					

Representative	Yea	Nay	Present	Representative	Yea	Nay	Present
Mr. Feenstra		X					
Ms. Malliotakis		X					
Mr. Carey		X					

In compliance with the Rules of the House of Representatives, the following statement is made concerning the vote of the Committee on Ways and Means during the markup consideration of H.R. 6918, the ''Supporting Pregnant and Parenting Women and Families Act'' on January 11, 2024.

The vote on the amendment offered by Mr. Davis to the amendment in the nature of a substitute to H.R. 6918, which would require that the legislation shall not take effect unless the Department of Health and Human Services submits a report to Congress on the total amount made available for part A of title IV of the Social Security Act provided to antiabortion centers and on the total number of applications for and recipients of assistance under State programs funded under such part to refer individuals to anti-abortion centers under or by such a program was not agreed to by a roll call vote of 17 yeas to 24 nays (with a quorum being present). The vote was as follows:

Representative	Yea	Nay	Present	Representative	Yea	Nay	Present
Mr. Smith (MO)		X		Mr. Neal	X		
Mr. Buchanan		X		Mr. Doggett	X		
Mr. Smith (NE)		X		Mr. Thompson	X		
Mr. Kelly		X		Mr. Larson	X		
Mr. Schweikert		X		Mr. Blumenauer	X		
Mr. LaHood		X		Mr. Pascrell	X		
Dr. Wenstrup		X		Mr. Davis	X		
Mr. Arrington		X		Ms. Sa´nchez	X		
Dr. Ferguson		X		Mr. Higgins	X		
Mr. Estes		X		Ms. Sewell	.		
Mr. Smucker		X		Ms. DelBene	X		
Mr. Hern		X		Ms. Chu	X		
Ms. Miller		X		Ms. Moore	X		
Dr. Murphy		X		Mr. Kildee	X		
Mr. Kustoff		X		Mr. Beyer	X		
Mr. Fitzpatrick				Mr. Evans	X		
Mr. Steube		X		Mr. Schneider	X		
Ms. Tenney		X		Mr. Panetta	X		
Mrs. Fischbach		X					
Mr. Moore		X					
Mrs. Steel		X					
Ms. Van Duyne		X					
Mr. Feenstra		X					
Ms. Malliotakis		X					

Representative	Yea	Nay	Present	Representative	Yea	Nay	Present
Mr. Carey		X					

In compliance with the Rules of the House of Representatives, the following statement is made concerning the vote of the Committee on Ways and Means during the markup consideration of H.R. 6918, the ‘‘Supporting Pregnant and Parenting Women and Families Act’’ on January 11, 2024.

The vote on the amendment offered by Ms. DelBene to the amendment in the nature of a substitute to H.R. 6918, which would prohibit the legislation from going into effect unless the Secretary of Health and Human Services finds there are no pregnancy center that provide misleading or deceptive information or puts at risk the health of women was not agreed to by a roll call vote of 18 yeas to 21 nays (with a quorum being present). The vote was as follows:

Representative	Yea	Nay	Present	Representative	Yea	Nay	Present
Mr. Smith (MO)		X		Mr. Neal	X		
Mr. Buchanan		X		Mr. Doggett	X		
Mr. Smith (NE)		X		Mr. Thompson	X		
Mr. Kelly		X		Mr. Larson	X		
Mr. Schweikert		X		Mr. Blumenauer	X		
Mr. LaHood		X		Mr. Pascrell	X		
Dr. Wenstrup		X		Mr. Davis	X		
Mr. Arrington				Ms. Sa´nchez	X		
Dr. Ferguson		X		Mr. Higgins	X		
Mr. Estes		X		Ms. Sewell	X		
Mr. Smucker		X		Ms. DelBene	X		
Mr. Hern		X		Ms. Chu	X		
Ms. Miller		X		Ms. Moore	X		
Dr. Murphy				Mr. Kildee	X		
Mr. Kustoff		X		Mr. Beyer	X		
Mr. Fitzpatrick				Mr. Evans	X		
Mr. Steube		X		Mr. Schneider	X		
Ms. Tenney		X		Mr. Panetta	X		
Mrs. Fischbach		X					
Mr. Moore							
Mrs. Steel		X					
Ms. Van Duyne		X					
Mr. Feenstra		X					
Ms. Malliotakis		X					
Mr. Carey		X					

In compliance with the Rules of the House of Representatives, the following statement is made concerning the vote of the Committee on Ways and Means during the markup consideration of H.R. 6918, the ''Supporting Pregnant and Parenting Women and Families Act,'' on January 11, 2024.

The vote on the amendment offered by Ms. Sewell to the amendment in the nature of a substitute to H.R. 6918, which would prohibit the legislation from going into effect unless the Secretary of Health and Human Services finds that all states have in effect laws that provide affordable access to healthcare for all women of reproductive age was not agreed to by a roll call vote of 18 yeas to 21 nays (with a quorum being present). The vote was as follows:

Representative	Yea	Nay	Present	Representative	Yea	Nay	Present
Mr. Smith (MO)		X		Mr. Neal	X		
Mr. Buchanan		X		Mr. Doggett	X		
Mr. Smith (NE)		X		Mr. Thompson	X		
Mr. Kelly		X		Mr. Larson	X		
Mr. Schweikert		X		Mr. Blumenauer	X		
Mr. LaHood		X		Mr. Pascrell	X		
Dr. Wenstrup		X		Mr. Davis	X		
Mr. Arrington				Ms. Sa´nchez	X		
Dr. Ferguson		X		Mr. Higgins	X		
Mr. Estes		X		Ms. Sewell	X		
Mr. Smucker		X		Ms. DelBene	X		
Mr. Hern		X		Ms. Chu	X		
Ms. Miller		X		Ms. Moore	X		
Dr. Murphy				Mr. Kildee	X		
Mr. Kustoff		X		Mr. Beyer	X		
Mr. Fitzpatrick				Mr. Evans	X		
Mr. Steube		X		Mr. Schneider	X		
Ms. Tenney		X		Mr. Panetta	X		
Mrs. Fischbach		X					
Mr. Moore							
Mrs. Steel		X					
Ms. Van Duyne		X					
Mr. Feenstra		X					
Ms. Malliotakis		X					
Mr. Carey		X					

In compliance with the Rules of the House of Representatives, the following statement is made concerning the vote of the Committee on Ways and Means during the markup consideration of H.R. 6918, the ''Supporting Pregnant and Parenting Women and Families Act,'' on January 11, 2024.

H.R. 6918 was ordered favorably reported to the House of Representatives as amended by a roll call vote of 24 yeas to 18 nays (with a quorum being present). The vote was as follows:

Representative	Yea	Nay	Present	Representative	Yea	Nay	Present
Mr. Smith (MO)	X			Mr. Neal		X	
Mr. Buchanan	X			Mr. Doggett		X	
Mr. Smith (NE)	X			Mr. Thompson		X	
Mr. Kelly	X			Mr. Larson		X	
Mr. Schweikert	X			Mr. Blumenauer		X	
Mr. LaHood	X			Mr. Pascrell		X	
Dr. Wenstrup	X			Mr. Davis		X	
Mr. Arrington	X			Ms. Sa´nchez		X	
Dr. Ferguson	X			Mr. Higgins		X	
Mr. Estes	X			Ms. Sewell		X	
Mr. Smucker	X			Ms. DelBene		X	
Mr. Hern	X			Ms. Chu		X	
Ms. Miller	X			Ms. Moore		X	
Dr. Murphy				Mr. Kildee.		X	
Mr. Kustoff	X			Mr. Beyer		X	
Mr. Fitzpatrick	X			Mr. Evans		X	
Mr. Steube	X			Mr. Schneider.		X	
Ms. Tenney	X			Mr. Panetta		X	
Mrs. Fischbach	X						
Mr. Moore	X						
Mrs. Steel	X						
Ms. Van Duyne	X						
Mr. Feenstra	X						
Ms. Malliotakis	X						

IV. Budget Effects of the Bill

A. Committee Estimate of Budgetary Effects

With respect to clause 3(d) of rule XIII of the Rules of the House of Representatives, a cost estimate provided by the congressional Budget Office pursuant to section 402 of the Congressional Budget Act of 1974 was not made available to the Committee in time for the filing of this report.

B. Statement Regarding New Budget Authority and Tax Expenditures Budget Authority

In compliance with clause 3(c)(2) of rule XIII of the Rules of the House of Representatives, the Committee states that the bill involves no new or increased budget authority. The Committee states further that the bill involves no new or increased tax expenditures.

V. Cost Estimate Prepared by the Congressional Budget Office

With respect to the requirements of clause 3(c)(2) of rule XIII of the Rules of the House of Representatives and section 308(a) of the Congressional Budget Act of 1974 and with respect to requirements of clause (3)(c)(3) of rule XIII of the Rules of the House of Representatives and section 402 of the Congressional Budget Act of 1974, the Committee has requested but not received a cost estimate for this bill from the Director of Congressional Budget Office. The Chairman of the Committee shall cause such estimate and statement to be printed in the Congressional Record upon its receipt by the Committee.

VI. Other Matters to Be Discussed Under the Rules of the House

A. Committee Oversight Findings and Recommendations

With respect to clause 3(c)(1) of rule XIII of the Rules of the House of Representatives, the Committee made findings and recommendations that are reflected in this report.

B. Statement of General Performance Goals and Objectives

With respect to clause 3(c)(4) of rule XIII of the Rules of the House of Representatives, the Committee advises that the bill does not authorize funding, so no statement of general performance goals and objectives is required.

C. Information Relating to Unfunded Mandates

This information is provided in accordance with section 423 of the Unfunded Mandates Reform Act of 1995 (Pub. L. No. 104–4). The Committee has determined that the bill does not contain Federal mandates on the private sector. The Committee has determined that the bill does not impose a Federal intergovernmental mandate on State, local, or tribal governments.

D. Congressional Earmarks, Limited Tax Benefits, and Limited Tariff Benefits

With respect to clause 9 of rule XXI of the Rules of the House of Representatives, the Committee has carefully reviewed the provisions of the bill, and states that the provisions of the bill do not contain any congressional earmarks, limited tax benefits, or limited tariff benefits within the meaning of the rule.

E. Duplication of Federal Programs

In compliance with clause 3(c)(5) of rule XIII of the Rules of the House of Representatives, the Committee states that no provision of the bill establishes or reauthorizes: (1) a program of the Federal Government known to be duplicative of another Federal program; (2) a program included in any report from the Government Accountability Office to Congress pursuant to section 21 of Public Law 111–139; or (3) a program related to a program identified in the most recent Catalog of Federal Domestic Assistance, published pursuant to the Federal Program Information Act (Pub. L. No. 95– 220, as amended by Pub. L. No. 98–169).

VII. Changes in Existing Law Made by the Bill, as Reported

In compliance with clause 3(e) of rule XIII of the Rules of the House of Representatives, the bill doesn't make any changes to existing law.

VIII. Dissenting Views

Committee on Ways and Means, House of Representatives,
Washington, DC, January 16, 2024.

DISSENTING VIEWS ON THE SUPPORTING PREGNANT AND PARENTING WOMEN AND FAMILIES ACT, H.R. 6918 H.R. 6918 doubles down on Republicans' extreme, unpopular war on women

Ways and Means Democrats strongly oppose H.R. 6918, which would allow states to divert funding intended for poor children to anti-abortion propaganda and facilities that provide deceptive and inaccurate information, endanger women's health with very little oversight, and put women's health in danger. This legislation does nothing to strengthen access to maternal health care, protect pregnant women, or increase federal support for struggling families.

The partisan bill, introduced by Rep. Fischbach, would permanently prevent the Department of Health and Human Services (HHS) from regulating state expenditure of Temporary Assistance for Needy Families (TANF) funding for so-called ''crisis pregnancy centers'' or anti-abortion centers (AACs). Under the bill, HHS would not be able to require data reporting, enforce statutory requirements, or prevent coercion or harm to low-income women for TANF-funded AACs.

AACs masquerade as health care facilities, usually providing misleading or inaccurate medical information in order to prevent women from seeking abortions. The recent HHS regulation this legislation would block notes that AACs target women who are already pregnant and therefore cannot reasonably meet TANF's purpose of reducing out-of-wedlock childbearing; thus, they should only receive funding if they meet other TANF purposes, including helping low-income children live with their parents, reducing use of government assistance, or promoting family formation.[11] Under the bill, AACs would be exempt from the requirement to meet TANF's statutory purposes, but pregnancy centers or other TANF-funded entities that did not have an explicit anti-abortion mission would be subject to regulation.

This is just another extremist bill from Republicans, timed to satisfy their anti-women base that is marching on Washington this week.

---

[11] Strengthening Temporary Assistance for Needy Families As a Safety Net and Work Program, 88 Fed. Reg. 67,697, Oct. 2, 2023.

Anti-abortion centers provide misleading information and should not receive federal taxpayer dollars.

Everyone deserves access to accurate information when making personal decisions. Anti-abortion centers (AACs)—sometimes referred to as Crisis Pregnancy Centers or CPCs—are not legitimate health care providers. They are organizations attempting to coerce pregnant people seeking abortions into carrying pregnancies to term through shame and misinformation. Pregnant people seeking pregnancy related counseling and services often find themselves at anti-abortion centers because of the deceptive way that these centers advertise themselves as legitimate, comprehensive health care providers. This bill would go further, allowing states to force low- income women to visit AACs in order to receive basic necessities like diapers.

Republicans rejected amendments to protect pregnant women from anti-abortion centers' deceptive, dangerous unlicensed medical practices.

During the Committee markup, extremist Republicans voted down amendments to prevent funding to organizations that deceived women about their purpose and qualifications or provided medically inaccurate information. Both amendments were rejected on a party line vote, despite recent cases in which women who went to so-called ''crisis pregnancy centers'' later had to seek emergency medical care because unqualified personnel missed ectopic pregnancies and other dangerous conditions. Republicans also refused to prevent coercive referrals of women who needed emergency financial assistance or basic necessities but were made to believe that they could only receive it if they gave up their reproductive rights.

Republicans voted against Democratic amendments to support pregnant women and mothers.

Despite the bill's misleading title about ''supporting'' pregnant women and families, extremist Republicans rejected amendments to ensure that families with poor children under 5 had food, housing, child care, and access to reproductive health care. Republicans also refused to require states to provide any data about how any diverted money was spent or demonstrate that women's health and economic futures were not being harmed.

AACs receive federal tax dollars to pursue an extremist ideological agenda at the expense of low-income mothers and children.

Comprehensive data does not exist, but using publicly available information, the watchdog group Equity Forward identified at least 10 states that had diverted funds intended to help poor children and families to fund anti-abortion organizations. Michigan[12] and Pennsylvania[13] have terminated their contracts, but Arkansas, Indiana, Louisiana, Missouri, North Carolina, North Dakota, Ohio, Oklahoma, and Texas are all thought to have current contracts providing such expenditures.[14] Eight of the nine states funding anti-abortion centers served less than 15 percent of poor families in their states, and two (Texas and Arkansas) served less than 5 per- cent of families in need.[15] In most states, the maximum TANF ben- efit for a single parent with one child is less than $400 a month.[16]

We urge our colleagues to join us in opposing H.R. 6918.

Sincerely,
Richard E. Neal,
Ranking Member.

Ranking Member Richard E. Neal Committee on Ways and Means Markup of H.R. 6918, Dissenting Views, Thursday, January 11, 2024

Happy New Year, Mr. Chairman, and to all of our Committee members. I echo the Chairman's sentiments—you will be missed, Congressman Ferguson. I wish you all the best in life's next chapter.

Turning to the legislation at hand, after the least productive session of Congress since the Great Depression, I had hoped we'd open the new session on a better note, working together to help the people we represent. Instead, I am gravely disappointed to see that, with today's agenda, the majority has all but farmed itself out to be an arm of the Trump re-election campaign. Look no further than his comments last night, where he bragged about stripping women

---

[12] Tara Murtha, Women's Law Project, Michigan Governor Defunds PA Based ''Crisis Pregnancy Center'' Chain Real Alternatives after Allegations of Misuse of Funds (October 1, 2019).

[13] Ivy DeJesus, Penn Live, Gov. Josh Shapiro Cuts Funding to ''Crisis'' Pregnancy Centers from State Budget (August 4, 2023).

[14] Rachel Wormer, Equity Forward, Mapping Deception: A Closer Look at How States' Anti-Abortion Center Programs Operate (September 2021).

[15] Aditi Shrivastava and Gina Azito Thompson, Center on Budget and Policy Priorities, TANF Cash Assistance Should Reach Millions More Families to Lessen Hardship (February 18, 2022).

[16] Gene Falk & Patrick A. Landers, Congressional Research Service, The Temporary Assistance for Needy Families (TANF) Block Grant: Responses to Frequently Asked Questions (February 27, 2023).

of their essential rights and freedoms. He called the end of Roe v Wade: "a miracle."

Next week, Washington will be the site of the largest anti-abortion rally in the country, and this legislation is to pander to attendees. Rather than listen to women about what they and their families need, or take action to address child poverty, the Majority has chosen to pursue another political talking point. What's worse, with this bill, they are choosing to divert money away from needy families to dangerous anti-abortion centers.

This isn't about health care or reproductive freedom or even their wildly unpopular anti-abortion agenda, it's fundamentally about control. Republicans have long been on a crusade to control and limit the rights of women.

Our Committee has work to do, and people depend on us to do so. We should be focused on addressing the maternal health crisis in this country, which is harming black women most of all.

This committee's mission is to safeguard health care, not attack it. After all, abortion care is health care, and it is overwhelmingly safe. But when health care is difficult or even impossible to access, that's when complications arise, and health outcomes worsen. We've seen horror after horror come out of Texas since their Republican governor and Supreme Court banned proper care.

Around the country, anti-abortion centers masquerading as health care providers are jeopardizing women's health and endangering their lives. In Massachusetts, one of these centers failed to correctly diagnose a woman's ectopic pregnancy because the staff wasn't qualified to be handling medical care. This misdiagnosis gravely endangered her life and necessitated emergency surgery a month later.

Furthermore, these centers aren't held to the same privacy or care standards as health providers.

This is not acceptable medical care, and it's horrifying that some of these propaganda centers are getting federal funding legally designated for serving poor children. This bill wants to fund more dangerous propaganda and more undeserving facilities of this kind. Women are being put in harm's way, their health is on the line, and it is all in the service of far-right ideology.

Beyond that, I'd be remiss if I didn't mention that we are only 9 days from another potential Republican government shutdown.

That's the fourth this Congress! Another damaging, but completely avoidable outcome for our economy and America's families.

Republicans are wasting precious time with political stunts like this one, which everyone in this room understands has zero chance of becoming law.

If Republicans wanted to pass legislation that lived up to the name of this bill, they could start by addressing the growing child care shortage caused by cutting off emergency child care funding and the enhanced dependent care tax credits that Democrats championed during the pandemic.

Or they could address the historic rise—a doubling—of child poverty caused by their refusal to extend the enhanced Child Tax Credit.

Or they could make paid family and medical leave a reality and spare struggling families from having to make the heartbreaking decision between caring for a loved one and losing a needed paycheck.

If you want to support parents, and support pregnant women, let's start by helping them, not misinforming them, criminalizing them, and making their lives harder.

With that, I yield back the balance of my time.

Richard E. Neal,
Ranking Member.

Chapter 12

Preparing for Your Baby: Information for Pregnant People with Substance Use Disorders[*,≠]

The U.S. Department of Health and Human Services

Congratulations on your pregnancy and getting ready for life with a new baby! Being a parent can be filled with great moments and challenges.

If you use alcohol or other drugs—or are in recovery—this is a time to think about how to best care for both of you.

If you are wondering what to expect while you are pregnant and after, this factsheet has information to help you make the best decisions.

You are not alone. Many people with substance use disorders (SUDs) or in recovery feel nervous upon learning they're pregnant. Fortunately, professionals who understand your needs can help! So can people who have lived through some of the same things you are dealing with right now.

Take steps toward treatment and recovery. If you're struggling with alcohol or other drug use—and aren't in treatment—it's important to find a good SUD treatment provider. Some communities have SUD treatment providers who focus on working with people who are pregnant or new parents. They understand your needs! If you are in SUD treatment or recovery, it's important to connect with a treatment provider or support group that understands pregnancy and parenting. Someone who has lived through some

---

[*] This is an edited, reformatted and augmented version of Substance Abuse and Mental Health Services Adminisration Publication.

[≠] This document uses the term "people" to be inclusive of women, nonbinary, transgender or non-conforming individuals experiencing pregnancy or in a parenting role.

In: Navigating Pregnancy Challenges
Editor: Javier Giles
ISBN: 979-8-89530-857-8

of the same things you are dealing with now, usually called a peer support, can be helpful.

You can also seek help through recovery support meetings, such as Alcoholics Anonymous, Narcotics Anonymous, and Self-Management and Recovery Training (SMART Recovery). You can find local SUD treatment and recovery support meetings by calling SAMHSA's National Helpline at 800-662-HELP (4357). This free, confidential service is available 24 hours a day.

How Could Alcohol and Other Drugs Affect My Baby?

- Substance Use While Pregnant and Breastfeeding
- Tobacco, Alcohol, Drugs, and Pregnancy
- Your Pregnancy and Substance Use

Common Substance Use Disorder Treatment Questions

What does treatment look like and how do I find it?

- Substance Abuse and Mental Health Services Administration (SAMHSA) Treatment Help Line and Treatment Locator Treatment Help Line and Treatment Locator
- SAMHSA Tip Sheet on Quality SUD Treatment

What is medication to treat substance use disorders/medication to treat opioid use disorder (MOUD) and can pregnant people use it?

- Treating Opioid Use Disorders in Pregnant Women

What if I need to go into residential treatment?

- SAMHSA Treatment Locator

Is there anyone who has done this before who can help me?

- SAMHSA Benefits of Peer Support in SUD Treatment and Recovery

Who will be on my SUD treatment team?

- As a pregnant women and pregnant people with a SUD, you may have many people on your care team. They can include a MOUD provider, home visitor, mental health therapist, peer support, clinical SUD counselor, and others who can help you with your mental and physical health needs and the needs of your baby.

How can I get treatment if I do not have transportation?

- SAMHSA Virtual Recovery Resources Listing

Getting to treatment and staying there isn't easy. You may worry about how alcohol or other drugs use may affect your pregnancy and your baby. These feelings, as well as concerns about how other people may react, can make it feel like you would rather not talk to anyone about it. But as reaching out for help with your alcohol or other drugs use is the first step to becoming a strong advocate for yourself and your baby. Getting treatment and attending all prenatal care visits ensure both of you receive the best possible start.

Pay attention to your feelings. You may feel down or worried during this time. These emotions are normal if they are mild and don't last long. For some people, pregnancy and new parenthood can make your feelings worse and even overwhelming. This may mean you have developed a mental health disorder. How do you know? Risk factors include a family history of depression, anxiety, bipolar, or other mental health disorders; a mental health disorder in a previous pregnancy; a history of trauma including intimate partner violence and abuse; and stressful life situations. Learn more about signs, symptoms, risk factors, and treatment for maternal mental health disorders at Maternal Mental Health Now. You can also use the SAMHSA Treatment Help Line and Treatment Locator to find mental health treatment available near you.

Many people can help. In addition to the treatment providers, there are many medical professionals who can help during and after your pregnancy. They may include

- An obstetrician/gynecologist (OB/GYN) who may deliver your baby and follow up afterwards to ensure both of you are healthy
- Labor and delivery nurses

- Hospital social workers who help you figure out what you need when you leave the hospital
- Other professionals who can help you and your baby stay safe and healthy

Choosing people for your team that you trust is important so that you feel safe sharing personal information about treatment, services, and needs. Your team is most helpful when they understand the needs of families affected by SUDs. Having a team that can speak up for you is important for all families. It's especially important for families of color who may have experienced bias, discrimination, and racism from the systems that provide them services. Good things can happen when your care team has plenty of information, talks openly, and knows you well!

Learn to care for your baby. If you used alcohol or other drugs during pregnancy, your baby may need some extra medical care after birth. If your baby is born with signs of substance withdrawal or other health-related issues, they may need to stay in the hospital longer. They may stay in a special nursery, a neonatal intensive care unit (NICU), or in the room with you. Time, love, and attention from their caregivers are a crucial part of caring for your new baby. The booklet Baby Steps explains how you, your family, and your care team can get off to a healthy start.

What's a "Plan of Safe Care"? Your care team may help you put together a Plan of Safe Care, or POSC, to organize information about the services you and your infant need, the people with whom you work, and what happens next. Some teams start this plan while you are pregnant while others wait until birth. Working on a POSC is a chance for you to gather input about what you both can expect next.

The POSC organizes information about available services and resources. It also helps you keep track of your team and enables them to share information to support you. Many plans also have checklists to remind you of important things to know before your baby goes home with you, such as where the baby will sleep, how to soothe infants when they are upset, how to properly install a car seat, where to reach out for help when experiencing challenges to your mental health, and how to access basic support like childcare, housing and food.

Why Is This Tool Called a Plan of Safe Care?

The federal government wants professionals who take care of pregnant women and pregnant people, their babies, and their families to make sure that infants with parents who used alcohol or other drugs have the necessary supports to be healthy. To that end, each state has to create "Plans of Safe Care" for families with babies who were born affected by a parent's use of alcohol or other drugs. While these plans may look a little different from state to state (and even town to town), they are supposed to include information about: 1) the services you need to be healthy, 2) the services your baby needs to be healthy, and 3) the things your family needs to thrive.

POSC also include information about which people and organizations are going to help you with each of those needs, and how they will make sure that you're getting what your family needs. You can find out more about the rules in your state here.

Child Welfare and Child Protective Services

How the Child Welfare System Works provides detailed information about the child welfare system, processes, and functions.

Contact With Child Welfare and Common Child Welfare Questions also includes information on child welfare cases specific to native families.

What are the laws about a parent using alcohol or other drugs in my state?

- Parents Substance Use as Child Abuse provides laws about a parent using alcohol or other drugs by state.

I'm not sure my child welfare case is going like it's supposed to. Can anyone help me?

Help with a Personal Issue Related to Child Welfare answers common child welfare question.

Learn how to work with child welfare. Many new parents wonder if child protective services, or CPS, will visit once their baby is born. When a newborn is born with alcohol or other drugs in their system, or a parent is identified as using substances, hospital staff contact CPS. CPS workers want to learn if the baby will be safe at home with their parent(s) and what might help your family stay healthy and safe. Sharing information with a CPS worker—including what you did to keep you and your infant healthy during your pregnancy and your participation in SUD treatment and prenatal care—helps them understand your situation. CPS workers will ask about these things to help them make recommendations for your infant's safety and well-being.

If a CPS worker determines you're not ready to fully care for your baby alone, they may recommend that: 1) both of you either live with someone who can support you in their care, or 2) your baby lives with someone else until you're ready. Continuing to participate in SUD treatment and other support services after your baby is born can help you stay focused on your POSC. Keeping that focus, even during this challenging time, remains important so that you can stay connected to your baby and reunify with him or her as quickly as possible.

Recovery is a lifelong process. When your baby is born—and during their first year—it's important to: 1) stay connected with your care team regularly, and 2) possibly include new people on that team. A peer support group (or person) could provide ongoing support. A recovery-friendly pediatric practice, which understands your unique needs as a parent in recovery and the special needs of your baby, could be a great asset to your care team.

A family support professional, such as an early intervention specialist, public health nurse, or home visitor can help you keep improving as a parent and understand if your baby is growing well. A mental health professional, such as a therapist or counselor, can check your mental health and watch for signs of postpartum depression (PPD). PPD can increase your risk of returning to substance use. It's important to talk with your care team about how you are feeling.

Your family can THRIVE! Pregnant women and pregnant and postpartum people along with their infants and families can—and do—successfully overcome these challenges.

Find Help with a Personal Situation

Substance Use and Mental Health Treatment Locator To find treatment facilities confidentially, 24/7 please call 1-800-4357 (HELP) or visit SAMHSHA's Treatment Services Locator

National Child Abuse Hotline

If you suspect a child has been harmed by abuse or neglect, please call 1-800-422-4453.

National Suicide Prevention Line For free and confidential support for people in distress, 24/7, please call or text 988, chat 988Lifeline.org, or call 1-800-273-8255.

Contact Us

This document is used as a supplement to Substance Abuse and Mental Health Services Administration's (SAMHSA) Clinical Guidance for Treatment and Parenting Women with Opioid Use Disorder and Their Infants.

To learn more about the information in this fact sheet from National Center on Substance Abuse and Child Welfare (NCSACW) email us at NCSACW@cffutures.org or call toll-free at 1-866-493-2758.

Acknowledgement: This resource is supported by contract number 75S20422C00001 from the Children's Bureau (CB), Administration for Children and Families (ACF), co-funded by the Substance Abuse and Mental Health Services Administration (SAMHSA). The views, opinions, and content of this brief are those of the authors and do not necessarily reflect the views, opinions, or policies of ACF, SAMHSA or the U.S. Department of Health and Human Services (HHS).

Chapter 13

Resources for Professionals Working with Pregnant and Parenting People Affected by Substance Use Disorders*,≠

The U.S. Department of Health and Human Services

Resource Title & Organization	Resource Description
Plans of Safe Care for Infants with Prenatal Substance Exposure and Their Families Child Welfare Information Gateway	Examines state laws and policies regarding the development and implementation of Plans of Safe Care (POSC)—as required by the Child Abuse Prevention and Treatment Act (CAPTA)—to ensure the safety and well-being of infants identified as being affected by prenatal substance use. Describes notification/reporting requirements; assessment of the infant and family; POSC development; services for the infant, parents, or other caregivers; and POSC monitoring.
Best Practices to Support Pregnant and Postpartum Women with Opioid Use Disorder and Infants Prenatally Exposed to Opioids Association of State and Territorial Health Officials and Centers for Disease Control	Describes best practices to support pregnant and postpartum women with opioid use disorder (OUD) and infants prenatally exposed to opioids. Featured topics include POSC, expanding access to OUD medications for pregnant and postpartum women, and using family-centered programs to treat OUD.

* This is an edited, reformatted and augmented version of The U.S. Department of Health and Human Services Publication.

≠ This document uses the term "people" to be inclusive of women, nonbinary, transgender or non-conforming individuals experiencing pregnancy or in a parenting role.

In: Navigating Pregnancy Challenges
Editor: Javier Giles
ISBN: 979-8-89530-857-8

Resource Title & Organization	Resource Description
Improving the Nurse-Family Partnership in Community Practice American Academy of Pediatrics	Specially trained registered nurses in the Nurse-Family Partnership (NFP) programs deliver home visits to first-time, low-income mothers for a period of 2½ years, lasting from early pregnancy until the child turns 2. This illustrated publication provides a framework to examine: 1) the NFP home-visiting model/implementation, and 2) promising approaches to challenges that may arise.
Pregnancy and Substance Use: A Harm Reduction Toolkit National Harm Reduction Coalition	Intended for pregnant and parenting people who use substances, along with their loved ones and service providers. Promotes the overall health and well- being of pregnant people who use substances. Many people, upon finding out they are pregnant, wonder about reducing or stopping their use. It is important to know there are many steps to take—related to substance use or not—toward a healthy pregnancy.
Maternal Mental Health Learning Opportunities for Providers Maternal Mental Health Now	Offers information on training, technical assistance, and other forms of consultation to health care and community-based providers serving families during their reproductive journey. The list includes therapists, clinical psychologists, social workers, community health workers, counselors, nurses (neonatal, pediatrics, labor and delivery, maternity, NICU), midwives, nurse practitioners, physicians (psychiatrists, OB/GYNs, pediatricians, neonatologists, family practitioners, general practitioners, primary care physicians), lactation consultants, health educators, doulas, and home visitors.
Mental Health of Parents and Caregivers Child Welfare Information Gateway	A parent or caregiver's mental health disorder can be a risk factor for child maltreatment. Depression, low self-esteem, poor impulse control, anxiety, and antisocial behavior are linked to a heightened potential for child abuse and neglect as these factors can compromise parenting. This resource list provides information on co-occurring mental health issues and child maltreatment.
Parental Substance Use as Child Abuse	Discusses laws and policies related to parental substance use, including the

Resource Title & Organization	Resource Description
Child Welfare Information Gateway	particular care and treatment needs of substance-exposed infants, risks to children, child neglect, and exposure to illegal drug activity. Contains full-text excerpts of laws for all U.S. states and territories.
Child Welfare Practice to Address Racial Disproportionality and Disparity Child Welfare Information Gateway	Examines racial disproportionality and disparity in child welfare and the factors that contribute to the problem. Also describes practices child welfare caseworkers, administrators, program managers, and policymakers can implement to assess these issues in general and at specific decision-making points along the child welfare continuum.
Addressing the Needs of Young Children in Child Welfare: Part C – Early Intervention Services Child Welfare Information Gateway	Describes the relationship between child welfare and early intervention (EI), provides an overview of the EI process, and outlines the challenges and strategies for implementing EI provisions in federal law. EI services can help young children (0-3) with developmental delays or disabilities—along with their families—overcome challenges and improve both well-being and outcomes. Partnerships between child welfare and EI systems can expand the array of supports and resources for all involved to help children remain safely in their homes, stabilize placements, and improve well-being.
Protective Factors Approaches in Child Welfare Child Welfare Information Gateway	Provides an overview of national protective factors approaches to prevent child abuse and neglect. Designed to help child welfare professionals, administrators, service providers, policymakers, and other interested individuals: 1) understand the concepts of protective and risk factors in families and communities, and 2) build protective factors to lower the risk of child abuse and neglect now and in the future.
The Indian Child Welfare Act: A Primer for Child Welfare Professionals Child Welfare Information Gateway	Provides caseworkers with an overview of current and historical issues affecting child welfare practice with American Indian and Alaska Native (AI/AN) families, practice implications, and cultural considerations. The

Resource Title & Organization	Resource Description
	1978 ICWA attempts to protect the right and culture of AI/AN children and families.
Substance Use, the Opioid Epidemic, and the Child Welfare System: Key Findings from a Mixed Methods Study U.S. Department of Health and Human Services, Office of the Assistant Secretary for Planning and Evaluation	Examines the relationship between parental substance use and child welfare caseloads, which began rising in 2012 after more than a decade of decline. Results describe how child welfare interacts with community partners to serve an increasing population of parents whose substance use has impaired their parenting and placed their children at risk.
How the Child Welfare System Works Child Welfare Information Gateway	Provides a brief overview of the purposes and functions of the child welfare system; offers a flowchart illustrating how cases typically move through the system.
How Federal Legislation Impacts Child Welfare Service Delivery Child Welfare Information Gateway	Provides an overview of the process by which legislative actions and policy changes at the federal level affect state and Tribal child welfare systems and service delivery; provides links to pertinent resources.
Alcohol Abuse and Other Substance Use Disorders: Ethical Issues in Obstetric and Gynecologic Practice The American College of Obstetricians and Gynecologists	Recommendations from the American College of Obstetricians on care for pregnant people with substance use disorders (SUDs). Includes routine screening techniques, clinical lab tests, brief interventions, and treatment referrals.
Opioid Use and Opioid Use Disorder in Pregnancy American College of Obstetricians and Gynecologists' and the American Society of Addiction Medicine	Provides ACOG recommendations on care for pregnant people with SUDs. Topics include universal screening for substance use as a comprehensive part of obstetric care, multidisciplinary long-term follow-up, infants born to women who used opioids during pregnancy, and referring pregnant people with OUDs to treatment to improve maternal and infant outcomes.
Family Engagement: Partnering with Families to Improve Child Welfare Outcomes Child Welfare Information Gateway	Overview of the foundational elements of the family engagement approach to child welfare as well as strategies and promising practices for implementing this approach. While geared toward frontline caseworkers who directly engage families, the publication also provides information about family engagement at the system, program, and community levels.
What is Child Welfare? A Guide for Health Care Professionals	Offers health care professionals an overview of child welfare and describes ways they can

Resource Title & Organization	Resource Description
Child Welfare Information Gateway	work together to promote better outcomes for children and families.
What is Child Welfare? A Guide for Behavioral and Mental Health Professionals Child Welfare Information Gateway	Overview of child welfare services. Describes how behavioral and mental health professionals can partner with child welfare to ensure children, youth, and families receive appropriate services that promote healthy functioning and well-being.

Contact Us

Email: ncsacw@cffutures.org
Website: ncsacw.acf.hhs.gov
Call: 866-493-2758

This document is used as a supplement to Substance Abuse and Mental Health
Services Administration's (SAMHSA) Clinical Guidance for Treatment and Parenting Women with Opioid Use Disorder and Their Infants.

To learn more about the information in this resource guide from National Center on Substance Abuse and Child Welfare (NCSACW) email us at NCSACW@cffutures.org or call toll-free at 1-866-493-2758.

Acknowledgment: This resource is supported by contract number 75S20422C00001 from the Children's Bureau (CB), Administration for Children and Families (ACF), co-funded by the Substance Abuse and Mental Health Services Administration (SAMHSA). The views, opinions, and content of this brief are those of the authors and do not necessarily reflect the views, opinions, or policies of ACF, SAMHSA or the U.S. Department of Health and Human Services (HHS).

Index

Q

R

S

Y